QUESTIONS AND ANSWERS
ON STUTTERING

Publication Number 629
AMERICAN LECTURE SERIES®

A Monograph in
AMERICAN LECTURES IN COMMUNICATION

Edited by
DOMINICK A. BARBARA, M.D., F.A.P.A.
Formerly Head, Speech Department
Karen Horney Clinic
New York, New York

QUESTIONS AND
ANSWERS
ON STUTTERING

By

DOMINICK A. BARBARA, M.D., F.A.P.A.

Certified Practicing Psychoanalyst
Associated with the American Institute for Psychoanalysis
Formerly Head, Speech Department
Karen Horney Clinic
New York, New York

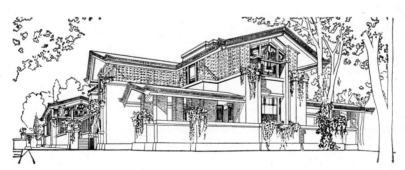

CHARLES C THOMAS • PUBLISHER
Springfield • Illinois • U.S.A.

Published and Distributed Throughout the World by

CHARLES C THOMAS • PUBLISHER

BANNERSTONE HOUSE

301-327 East Lawrence Avenue, Springfield, Illinois, U.S.A.

NATCHEZ PLANTATION HOUSE

735 North Atlantic Boulevard, Fort Lauderdale, Florida, U.S.A.

*With THOMAS BOOKS careful attention is given to all details of
manufacturing and design. It is the Publisher's desire to present books
that are satisfactory as to their physical qualities and artistic possibilities
and appropriate for their particular use. THOMAS BOOKS will be true
to those laws of quality that assure a good name and good will.*

Printed in the United States of America

A-2

PREFACE

This small book is a serious attempt to bring together most of the important facts and theories known today about stuttering. In the form of short, simple and concise questions and answers, problems pertinent to this baffling subject are presented for the interested professional and lay person. In its pages the reader will find some of these specific questions answered:

1. What Is Stuttering?
2. Is Stuttering Inherited?
3. How Does Stuttering First Manifest Itself?
4. What Theories Are There About Stuttering?
5. What Are the Family Backgrounds of Stutterers?
6. What Kind of Home Environment Can Lead to Stuttering?
7. What Are the Psychological Sources that Lead to Stuttering?
8. What Can Be Done to Prevent Stuttering?
9. Is There a Specific Age at Which Treatment of the Stuttering Child Should Begin?
10. Can Hypnotism Cure Stuttering?
11. How Are Adults Who Stutter Helped in Treatment?
12. Does Group Therapy Help in Stuttering?
13. What Is the Role of the Pediatrician and the Family Physician in the Handling of the Stuttering Problem?

Finally, this book can be invaluable as a text to beginning students in speech pathology, speech therapists, speech teachers, psychologists, psychiatrists and especially to stut-

vi   QUESTIONS AND ANSWERS ON STUTTERING

terers themselves and their families. It can be most bene-
ficial to pediatricians and general practitioners who have
to deal with the parents of the child and adolescent stutterer and who must prepare a general regimen of therapy
for the stutterer himself.

CONTENTS

QUESTIONS AND ANSWERS
ON STUTTERING

Chapter 1

COMMON FACTS AND CHARACTERISTICS CONCERNING STUTTERING

Let Us Begin by Asking, What Is Stuttering?

According to most dictionaries and the general public, stuttering is defined as "hesitating or stumbling in uttering words." To the speech therapist, however, this definition is not complete unless it is qualified by at least three statements: 1) the speaker has no discernable physical or mental abnormality that is functionally related to the hesitant speech; 2) he regards his way of speaking as unusual and considers it a problem or a difficulty, and 3) he seeks to contend with this difficulty by means of avoidance reactions that interfere with his speech.

Are Stuttering and Stammering the Same?

Stuttering and stammering are often used interchangeably. According to the derivation, stuttering stands for labored, difficult, hesitant speech with resultant defective conversation. Stammering, instead, refers to defects of articulation and should never be confused with stuttering. Stammering depends on performance, stuttering depends on emotional disturbances.

What Is the Incidence of Stuttering?

The incidence of stuttering amounts to about 1,500,000 in this country alone, 15,000,000 in the world. It has been placed at about 1 per cent of the general population, roughly half of whom are children. Stuttering has no respect for social or economic status, religion, race or intelligence.

What Are Some Characteristics About the Actual Symptom of Stuttering Itself?

No two stutterers perform their stuttering in exactly the same way, and any one stutterer varies somewhat in manner of performance during any given day, or hour, and from week to week and year to year.

Relating to the actual content of the stuttering itself, we find that 10 per cent of words are stuttered, the other 90 per cent are normal. Most stutterings last one or two seconds or less, and that repetition of initial sounds, prolongation of initial sounds, or exaggerated hesitancy to speak are common.

Finally, most stuttering occurs on words that are nouns, verbs, adjectives, and adverbs; that begin sentences; that are longer than the average word; and that begin with consonants rather than vowels.

Is Stuttering Inherited?

There is no organic proof of stuttering being inherited, although we do know that there is a familial tendency. Stuttering does run in families more often than in those of non-stutterers. Studies have found that over 65 per cent of patients who stuttered show a family history of stuttering. Other familial characteristics included relatively high incidence in twins and in family history of twins, relatively high incidence of left-handedness and ambidexterity, and slowness of speech development.

Are There Constitutional Factors Which Might Lead to Stuttering?

Despite the lack of any strong evidence pertaining to the causative factors in stuttering, there is some suggestion of the presence of constitutional factors which predispose an individual to emotional imbalance in general and to stuttering speech in particular. There also appears to be some predisposition in people who stutter to an original motor disorganization, since stuttering children are observed to be more awkward and less adept at acquiring motor skills than other children.

What Significance Is There in the Family History of Stutterers?

It was usually found, in most every case studied, that one or both parents were nervous, tempermental, worrisome, emotionally unstable, hypersensitive about speech, conscious of words, obsessive-compulsive in nature, fearful, presented psychosematic correlations in diseases of the upper respiratory and digestive systems, and also of ulcers, migraines and diseases of the cardiovascular system, pointing to inner tension.

How Does Stuttering First Manifest Itself?

Stuttering usually begins between the ages of two and six. Its development is progressive, beginning with a *clonic* spasm or block that causes excessive repetition of sounds, for example, M-m-m-m-m-Mummy. However, attention is soon called to his speech, so that he now tries to consciously keep from stuttering. At this secondary stage, the block begins to become *tonic,* with a prolonged fixation in speech production resulting in prolongation on initial sounds, for example, M mmmmmmmm Mummy. Neither tonic or clonic is a spasm in the strict medical sense, for it is thought to be voluntary rather than involuntary.

Why Are There More Males Than Females Who Stutter?

Males are from four to eight times as frequently affected than females. One explanation for this, I believe, is that early environmental stress is never as hard on girls as on boys. The element of social competition enters into the life of even the youngest boys much more decisively than into that of girls. For, the little girls play with each other in groups, the same as they did when they played with their mothers or sisters at home, while the boy is injected immediately into an incomparably more strenuous atmosphere of group games in which the prowess of much older boys sets the standards. In other words, the social impact is stronger in the male sex and stuttering, therefore, must be more common. Also, an additional hardship for the male is the fact that mothers usually center their affection on him (injudiciously) shielding him and thereby weakening him, with the result that he is unable to cope with the regular environmental onslaughts.

Are There Fixed Personality Components Between Males and Females Which Might Affect the Ratio of Stutterers?

Yes, according to Dr. Allen of the Mayo Clinic, the fixed personality components show decided differences. Dr. Allen tabulated over three hundred thousand cases and found that females are stronger and healthier than males. They showed in many ways greater psychological and neurological stability. Their susceptibility to many conditions was decidedly less pronounced than that of the male. And as he puts it, "the male is inferior to the female, and speaking comparatively, the price of maleness is weakness." This, in a way, is a definite reflection on their ability to maintain normal control of all organs including speech organs. In fact, the female speech apparatus is stronger as well as more perfected in action, thus making for the development of a single neuromuscular pattern. As Dr. Allen well puts it: "Since the ability to speak is the result of training and girls are more loquacious, practicing speech all the time, it follows that with their finer mechanism, higher rhythmic sense, and better coordination, they are less liable to lose their balance under new environmental conditions."

Are More Boys Than Girls Referred to Speech and Reading Clinics?

More boys than girls are referred to clinics for speech retardation, special language disabilities, and articulatory speech defects. Approximately three times as many boys as girls are referred to clinics for reading disabilities. Boys make more errors than girls in writing and spelling, and their school achievement correlates well with their intelligence. At the pre-school and elementary school level, sex differences in intelligence and school achievement, as determined by standard tests, by grade status, and teachers' ratings consistently favor girls rather than boys. The difference in achievement is reversed at the high school level by the addition of courses in science, mathematics, and social studies, in which boys tend to excel, but girls tend to maintain their superiority in language.

What Relative Importance Does the Factor of Imitation Play in Stuttering?

There is no doubt the factor of imitation of necessity enters into the total picture and may add to the problem itself in the long run. A child in its early years may imitate a stuttering parent, or, in a playful sense, imitate a stuttering child. However, this will not be of lasting effect in the final analysis unless many more complex factors have entered into the same situation and speech consciousness, therefore, becomes more prevalent. To say that one can acquire stuttering by imitation alone, I feel, has very little basis. Stuttering can, and will, develop in a tense and worrisome home which would ordinarily lead to emotional inadequacy and where there is an added factor of an over-emphasis on difficult speech.

Does a Parent's Insisting That a Child Change from Left-handedness to Using His Right Cause Stuttering?

Although left-handedness and stuttering quite often do occur together, most specialists agree that the changing handedness is not a direct cause of stuttering. What can be of more serious detriment to the child's security and emotional balance, however, is the effect of anything in the family situation that might tend to make him feel different and rejected by his parents. If parents constantly make an issue of the child's left-handedness, anxieties are produced that may interfere with the calmness and relaxation necessary to fluency in speech. Such are the possible indirect connections between stuttering and left-handedness. It is, therefore, not wise for parents to interfere with the natural handedness of the child, but to do so does not directly cause stuttering.

Why Do Most Stutterers Not Stutter When They Sing?

Swift, in his imagery theory, postulates that a person who stutters has no trouble when he sings because the melody area in the brain takes the prominent part in the control of the speech utterances while in regular speech the usual area functions as the main control.

I personally feel that since our society is speech-conscious, and since communication and verbalization tend to be overemphasized, the act of speaking in itself becomes identified with competition, prestige, and success. However, we do not place the same demands or stresses upon ourselves when we sing, the latter being identified rather with pleasure and relaxation. In consequence, there is bound to be much more anxiety and apprehension tied up with speaking than there is with singing.

Is Stuttering a Complex Problem?

Stuttering is a highly complex syndrome. It has a multiple etiology, and has often, and properly, been called the disorder of many theories. Specialists in practically every field of speech and medical research, seeking to cope with this problem according to their own individual findings, have but added to the complexity and confusion. Only by approaching the problem from a dynamic and holistic point of view, and keeping in mind that we are treating not solely a "voice disorder," but a total human being, can we hope to understand its nature. To be effective, this approach must concern itself with the affliction less as a speech disturbance and more as a manifestation of the feelings, attitudes, and responses implicit in the actual speaking situation.

Does Stuttering Date Back to Ancient Times?

The problem of stuttering was recorded by the ancients. Aristotle, Hippocrates, Galen, and Celsus all theorized about the causes of stuttering and proposed remedies for its cure, among them the use of healing oils, cauterization of the tongue, and breathing exercises. World famous figures who were stutterers included Moses, Aristotle, Aesop, Demosthenes, Virgil, Charles I, Charles Lamb, Charles Darwin, and, in modern times, Sir Winston Churchill, W. Somerset Maugham, and George VI.

How Do Present-day Theorists Feel About Stuttering?

Until about fifty years ago, stuttering was understood only slightly and practically never remediable. Its cause was thought to be physical, its nature was erroneously described, and its treatment often involved radical surgery, usually with tragic consequences. Today, although no one has yet discovered the actual underlying cause of stuttering, a great deal more is known about factors contributing to its development. Where the tongue was once the chief organ of choice, today the organicity is attributed mainly to the more complicated neurophysiological aspects of the entire speech tract.

Finally, in the struggle toward arriving at a clearer understanding toward the problem of stuttering, there are those researchers who attempt to attribute psychological factors to its *modus operandi*. These latter theoreticians seem to be gaining supporters and the most sympathetic and interested audience in the field of speech pathology.

What Is the Psychogenic Theory for Stuttering by Dr. Barbara?

This theory is based chiefly on findings of considerably more signs of maladjustment in stutterers than in nonstutterers. The stuttering is described as an expression of anxiety in an insecure individual when his psychological barriers are threatened and disorganized. Where the stutterer differs from other neurotic individuals is in the special attitudes, feelings, and beliefs relevant to his particular neurotic development and to the expression of these conflicts specifically in the "speaking situation." The stutterer is, therefore, seen as a human being suffering from neurotic difficulties which are expressed overtly when he speaks and especially so at the time of stuttering. Only by working with his whole personality, according to Doctor Barbara, will the stutterer be able to find real inner balance, healthy coordination of all his feelings and actions—including that of relaxed and spontaneous speech.

What Is the Conditioned Response Theory to Stuttering?

The late Dr. C. S. Bluemel believed that speech is a conditioned response and that stuttering is an inhibition which occurs before the speech reflex is securely established. Stuttering has its onset in the early years of life because the conditioned reflex of speech is not yet stable. On the other hand, stuttering rarely begins in adult life, because the conditioned reflex of speech is now a fixed and secure response.

What Is the Freudian Explanation for Stuttering?

According to Doctor Coriat, "Stuttering is a psychoneurosis caused by the persistence into later life of early pregenital oral nursing, oral sadistic, and anal sadistic components. The term 'pregenital' refers to the organization of the sexual life of the child during the early infantile period before the genital zone has assumed a dominating role. In cases of stuttering, these various pregenital tendencies can't be definitely observed when attempts are made to speak and they also appear in characteristic oral nursing and oral cannibalistic dreams, showing that the stutterer has not overcome these pregenital impulses in the course of adult development."

Describe the Cerebral Dominance Theory for Stuttering?

The cerebral dominance or handedness theory is based on the neurologic fact that the right side of the body is controlled by the left side of the brain and vice versa. Since the organs of speech lie along the midline of the body and consist of paired muscles governed by different hemispheres of the brain, the idea was advanced that any inharmony of action occurring in the brain may upset muscular coordination of the speech organs. This idea was also supported by the finding that many stutterers are left-handed, and that many of them were forced to use the right hand, producing central disturbance of cerebral dominance. However, it does not explain stuttering in right-handed stutterers or those left-handed ones who were never forced to change to right-handedness. Moreover, it has shown that lack of motor coordination in stutterers is not related to handedness.

What Theory Favors "Learned Behavior" as an Explanation for Stuttering?

A group of investigators at the University of Iowa Speech Clinic favor the theory that stuttering is learned behavior. Stuttering begins at an age when most children normally repeat forty to fifty times per 1,000 words spoken. Over-anxious parents mistake normal repetitions and hesitations for stuttering, and try to make the child speak "correctly." Parents insist that the child "speak slowly" or "stop and start again;" they reprimand or even punish him. This kind of parent has probably created tension and anxiety in other spheres as well. In an attempt to win approval, the child tries to change his speech by holding his breath, clamping his jaws, and compressing his lips. Says Johnson, "But these things he does to 'keep himself from stuttering' are exactly the stuttering he is trying to avoid. In this sense, then, the harder the stutterer tries to keep from stuttering the more things he does that we call stuttering."

Finally, What Theory Favors a Disturbance of the Thought Processes as a Cause for Stuttering?

Froeschels calls stuttering "dissociative aphasia." He believes that there is a disturbance of the thought processes, a deficiency in word finding and sentence formation and, later on, an interference between the ideas which the patient wants to utter and ideas of existing difficulties. At the onset, the causes are largely physiological in nature (because about 80 per cent of children pass through a short period of syllable-repeating), but, as time passes, psychological reactions develop which may be considered a form of psychoneurosis. Froeschels finds considerable evidence that the affliction is linked up with subconscious volition, the will to stutter.

Chapter 2

THE DEVELOPMENT OF STUTTERING IN THE YOUNG CHILD

Do All Children Go Through a Stage of Hesitant and Repetitive Speech?

To say that all children "go through a stage" in which they speak hesitantly and repetitiously is not quite true. According to Wendell Johnson, "repetition starts with the birth cry—which consists practically always of the vowel 'a' as in 'hat,' repeated several times — and continues throughout infancy. It does not miraculously stop when the child begins to say words. It does decrease gradually with increasing age, other things being equal, but there is no day, hour, or minute in life when it suddenly ceases altogether. There is really no 'stage' that the child goes through. It is simply that speech follows a course of development. Throughout this course there is non-fluency, although the relative amount of it decreases noticeably from infancy to adulthood."

Are All Parents Aware of Their Children's Hesitations?

No, in fact in most homes, particularly those in which no one has had any personal experience with stuttering, the normal non-fluency of beginning speech is almost completely disregarded. Most parents in this instance, are surprised to learn that the average child repeats forty-five times per thousand words. They do not remember any repeating or hesitations to speak of.

In homes where children are permitted to develop their own individual speech, with all its normal non-fluencies, and without being made self-conscious about it by parents who are overly concerned and perfectionistic—there is no stuttering. However, the reverse occurs in those parental settings where the basic attitudes and beliefs are those of apprehension, worry and overconcern about the child as a whole, including his speech.

Should a Parent Be Unduly Concerned About a Child's Hesitant Speech?

One should certainly not be concerned about normal non-fluency. This is immature speech or non-organized speech; it is speech in the making, which is normal to childhood.

It is important during this period for parents to avoid an anxious and obsessive attitude toward a child's speech. The child must not feel that he is different or abnormal, and that his speech is something in which he is found to be deficient. If he stutters, he should not be corrected with such admonitions as "Slow down, say it again," "Say it nicely," "Don't stutter," etc. In fact, the child's speech difficulties should be played down, while his physiological and psychological needs should be played up. A child may be praised for good speech in an assuring way, but not in a manner that implies anxiety for other occasions when speech is less fluent.

Do Children Tend to Stutter Following Certain Periods?

Children display stuttering during stress-filled periods such as during Christmas week, after picnics and parties, after busy weekends, after attending summer camp—in fact after any activity that leaves them tired and emotionally over-wrought.

During this time, a balance is essential between pleasurable activity and necessary rest. A stimulating day may call for a mild bedtime sedative, the "morning-after" might well be spent in bed, and when there is a definite tendency to disorganization, the child is usually benefited by a few extra hours of rest or sleep on Saturday and Sunday mornings. During this period of disorganization, we include not only stuttering, but also nervousness, irritability, loss of appetite, sleeplessness, nightmares, bedwetting, etc.

Do Repetitions or Hesitations in a Child Learning to Speak Constitute Stuttering?

The developmental hesitations of a child learning to speak are not stuttering—and from this viewpoint stuttering is not just nonfluency or hesitant, repetitious or unsmooth speech.

Beginning speech is normally quite non-fluent. The average child aged two to six years repeats about forty-five times per thousand words. He repeats sounds, or parts of words, like th-th-this; or whole words, like like like this; or phrases like this like this like this. He also participates in other types of hesitancies, stallings, 'um's,' 'ah's,' etc. All this is perfectly normal.

What Then Are the Signs of Beginning Stuttering?

It is vitally important that parents recognize the differences between stuttering and the normal hesitancies which all children show occasionally.

In a booklet published by the Speech Foundation of America, the following kinds of behavior are mentioned as deserving a calm concern:-

1) The child begins to show marked and obvious speech hesitancies;

2) He begins to avoid verbal contacts or becomes excessively shy about speaking in certain situations which he had formerly entered eagerly. The same holds true when this reluctance to speak involves a certain person;

3) He begins to speak with effort and strain, and is clearly struggling to express things which previously he had said easily;

4) Volleys of repetition of syllables or sounds, or the drawing out of sounds, begin to reappear more often.

Can a Parent's Improper Evaluation of These Early Hesitancies Affect a Child's Future Speech Pattern?

There is little doubt that if speech begins normally, stuttering is usually prevented.

Free-flowing and spontaneous speech in a child occurs mostly in an environment of parental warmth, freedom, and one in which the child feels accepted. Hesitancies in talking, however, first begin to express themselves in response to a parental setting of prohibitions and restitutions. This nonfluent speech and hesitancy in younger children may be normal to some degree, yet tense, overworried, and perfectionistic parent may tend to look at this as stuttering. Once the child has been labeled as a stutterer, his position again becomes unique, in that there is set in motion a chain reaction of worries, anxieties, and preoccupations, which gravely perturbs both child and parent.

What Kind of a Home Environment Can Usually Lead to Stuttering?

A child's hesitancies in speech are for the most part aggravated in parent-child situations which interfere with the normal expression of thought, feeling, and action. In a home in which there is an overemphasis on perfectionistic standards and regimes, there may well be present attitudes conducive to disapproval of nonfluent speech. A perfectionistic parent may compel his child to speak perfectly clearly and loudly. If the child talks slowly, words are practically taken out of his mouth, or interpreted for him. He may be constantly criticized for hesitating before starting to speak, and, when he finally does, for not saying the right words to begin with. He is taught to feel that words must be carefully chosen, that he must articulate perfectly clearly and master his communications. He must not falter or hesitate too long—must be brief about what he has to say and yet at the same time be prepared to say whatever may be expected of him at any time. Some perfectionistic parents may even go so far as to suggest other methods of talking which they feel will be better or easier for the child. These latter suggestions may include showing the child how to inhale before speaking and exhale afterward, to substitute other words for the more difficult ones whenever a hesitancy may occur, or to exercise willpower and to push speech, even though the child may be fatigued or excited. Parents of this sort will generally lose their own patience in the use of some of these rigid compulsions of theirs, and finally resort to some form of punishment, ridicule, or even sadistic embarrassment of the child in the presence of others.

What Role Does an Over-protective Parent Play in the Early Development of a Child's Speech?

The overprotective parent makes as many demands and expectations in her child's beginning speech development as the perfectionistic one. In this setting, however, the attitudes are usually camouflaged with a facade of over-concern, worry, and a persistent state of preoccupation.

The child, because of the overemphasis on being protected, is made to feel dependent upon his parent for constant approval, praise, and recognition, each time he expresses himself. He is taught to develop attitudes in what he is supposed to say, each time he opens his mouth. His speech, as a result of this overprotectiveness, is not experienced as being his own, but as coming from the outside, usually identified with his mother. He learns to mimic and imitate his mother in almost every way: "Mommy says don't do this, say this, eat this, watch out, be careful," etc. When he talks, he is driven to adhere to strict parental activities concerning *"what to say, how to say it,* and *when to say it."*

Most overprotective parents feel that their children should be "seen but not heard." They should never intrude when "Mommy" is talking, should have good manners, and should keep absolutely quiet when others are present. These same parents may listen quite attentively to their children when they feel it necessary, yet show very little consistent real interest or attention when needed. A child in such a prohibitive environment develops a fear and apprehension of talking. He becomes afraid of what will happen to him if he should talk at the wrong time, or say something that may not meet with his parents approval. These worrisome and anxious reactions in the parental setting sent into motion a circle of chain reactions which become of traumatic consequence to the child's further speech development.

How Does a Stuttering Child Perceive His Parents?

A child who stutters usually has ambivalent feelings of overt dependency mixed with deep underlying hostility which he is unable to express. He tends to see his mother as the domineering and controlling parent. He verbalizes such projections as: "My mother never gives me a chance to talk or to express myself. She thinks she is always right," "Most mothers are smotherers," "I like my mother, but I wish she wouldn't always nag me, and would leave me alone." Some stutterers, feeling freer to express their hostility, remarked, "My mother is a tyrant," "My mother is hell," "she is ruining my whole life." During these instances of open hostility, the stuttering usually lessened to a minimum.

While the stutterer sees his mother as being predominately possessive, he perceives his father as distant; far removed from him emotionally. He longs for a closer relationship with the person by whom he especially feels rejected. He feels that his father rarely thinks of him or understands him. He secretly wishes that his father were proud of him, would appreciate his problems, and be the master in the house.

How Does the Stuttering Child View Himself?

The stutterer views himself in many instances as not being an integral part of the family. He feels, rather, as an individual who is constantly being reacted to by the other family members. He senses that he is being disapproved of, criticized, blamed, or critically observed. He feels generally that he is perceived as being inept, immature, and as someone who is not capable of handling his own affairs. Toward his mother, he senses a great deal of hostility, which he is afraid to overtly express, and is guilty about these feelings. He finds she is too possessive, very superficial, of inferior intellect, too verbal, and desirous of controlling the male.

How Does a Stutterer Feel in Relationship to Others?

In respect to others, stutterers feel quite isolated and relatively incapable of developing mature relationships. From early childhood, they want very much to develop a closeness with people, but at the same time, there is the awareness that they have a problem in communicating with others verbally and emotionally. Associated with the desire for proximity with people is a definite hostility, the ambivalence making for much anxiety and stuttering. In the presence of others, they usually complain of feeling inadequate, victimized, inferior, and criticized to the point that makes communication a most difficult and threatening task.

Give 4 Brief Illustrations of Parental Settings Where Stuttering Might Occur.

The following are brief case studies of parental settings in stutter-type environments:*

Case 1
Johnny's family on both sides were of German-Polish descent, middle class. He is an only child born through a forced marriage due to an illegitimate pregnancy. His mother is a large, heavy-set, domineering, and perfectionistic individual. In her own family constellation, she played a minor role, being constantly oppressed and pushed into the background by her own mother and older sister, who was the family favorite. Johnny's father played instead a detached, aloof, and indifferent role, succumbing many times to his wife's demands in order to avoid too many arguments or friction. As a boy, Johnny was in constant fear of being punished in not being able to live up to his mother's absolute and perfectionistic demands. She exposed him to a domineering form of overprotection, as she dictated and charted every possible move he took. Onset of stuttering began at the age of nine.

---

*Case reports taken from author's book: *Stuttering: A Psychodynamic Approach to its Understanding and Treatment,* Julian Press, N. Y., 1954.

Case 2

Tony was born in a poorer Italian section of Brooklyn in 1927. Both parents were Italian, born in Sicily; they had migrated to this country because of social and economic goals. Tony was the only boy in a family of five older sisters. There were eight pregnancies in all, two of them ending in miscarriages. Tony's father felt angered and hostile each time his wife gave birth to a female child. He would rage at her for her incapacity to bear worthwhile children, and felt insignificant as a male in the eyes of his relatives and neighbors. He is further described as being aggressive, domineering, controlling and as an arrogant, vindictive tyrant. Because of his own cultural background, he strongly held to the dogma of male superiority. When Tony was born, his father shut his barber shop for a week and the home became a temple of worship and festivity. His "Christ-like" son had been born, and no longer had he to hang his head in shame and humiliation. Tony's mother, on the other hand, is described as being self-sacrificing, oversolicitous, and martyrlike in her suffering role. Tony's life had been charted and dictated ever since his birth: he was to become a successful doctor, lawyer, or dentist. The intense pressure of the unattainable goals forced upon Tony from an early age resulted in his beginning to stutter at the age of eight.

Case 3

Robert was born in New York, in 1922. The family on both sides was of Russian-Jewish descent, middle class. His mother is described as a small, aggressive, domineering, and controlling individual who assumed the dominant role in her own marriage. In her own family constellation, however, she played a minute role, being the only girl of a family of four siblings. In this family setting of hers, she felt as though she had to constantly assert herself in order to survive. She is further described as being extremely touchy, sensitive, suspicious, exploitative, and living under false pretenses of being lovable, honest, and sincere. Robert's father is described as being detached, shy, withdrawn, and a retiring person, who had little time for himself or his children. Toward him, his wife was constantly complaining, nagging, and belittling. After constant quarrels and bitter friction, Robert's father deserted his family and his whereabouts were unknown. This left his wife with all the more justification to feel embittered and abused. She was now compelled to go to work, and into the household came her own mother, which complicated the situation all the more. As a child, Robert was sickly and fragile. His mother felt guilty as a result of this and exposed him to a morbid form of overprotection. She constantly watched over him, showered him with gifts, embraced him affectionately whenever he conformed to her expectations, yet raged when he rebelled. She accompanied him to and from school, chose his friends, and was constantly in fear that he would hurt himself or get sick. Robert was rarely permitted to go out to play with the other children and was not allowed to partake in vigorous competitive sports. His mother would rule him with an iron hand, yet at times shower him with gifts, overaffection, and false love. As a result of this constant ambivalence of emotion, Robert felt persistent confusion, doubt, and apprehension. Stuttering began at the age of seven.

Case 4

Carmine was also born in a poorer section of Brooklyn, in 1926. His parents were of Italian-Irish descent, middle class. The family environment was one of constant arguments and friction over money matters, in-laws, and religious issues. The father was a severe stutterer who drank habitually, during which times he would beat his wife unmercifully in the presence of his son. During his wife's second pregnancy, he brutally kicked her abdomen, causing her to abort. When

Carmine was four years old, his father was killed in a street brawl during a drinking spree. Following this unfortunate event, Carmine's mother began to center all her energies and resources toward living vicariously through her son. She overprotected him and held him close to her apron strings. She went to work, boarded him with a neighbor of hers, and made up her mind never to marry again. She prayed and believed that her son would magically give her everything she wished for and of which she had been so cruelly and unjustly deprived. Carmine was her "baby," her only salvation toward peace and tranquillity. She guarded her precious possession with every ounce of her strength, and watched him grow with fear, apprehension, and selfish protectiveness. He started to stutter at the age of six.

Is a Stuttering Child's Position in a Family Unit Made to Be Unique, Special, or Different from Most Other Children's Environments?

For the most part it is. Factors which lead to this sort of a precarious position in the family setting result from some of the following basic sources: 1) The child predisposed to stuttering is usually an only child in a family unit. This may come about as a definite choice in a selfish, sacrificing mother or realistically following a separation, a divorce, or the death of one of the parents, usually the father. 2) His position can become predominant as a result of his being the only male child in a family of two or more females. 3) From deeply imbedded traditional cultural factors found in some parents of children who stutter. Many of these children are from families of minority groups—Italians, Jews, Negroes, Poles, etc.—where the cultural milieu gives importance to the special meaning of the male preference, the first son, or the first-born. Stress is also placed on the social importance of male superiority to female inferiority.

What are Some Basic Prerequisites for Healthy Development in a Child?

Although there are essential similarities in the growth patterns of individuals, no two children, even those in the same family constellation, are alike, either in themselves or in the way that they move through this sequence of development. Each child, when born, has his own moods, temperaments, potentialities, gifts, and his own particular capacities. In this same context, each individual child has his own physical, mental, and emotional attributes. A child afflicted at birth with some organic defect will most likely have a greater difficulty in adjusting and progressing through the periods of development than a more fortunate physically healthy one. In addition, cultural and economic factors at the time of birth also play an important role in the future developmental growth of the child.

Given the chance and a more or less healthy soil, a child can grow to become apparently normal and fulfill his growth possibilities. Basically, the soil must contain a feeling of genuine warmth, love and respect. A child needs to feel that his environment is one in which he is wanted, loved, needed, and one in which there is a sense of belonging. If this feeling is lacking, then a state of emotional stirring is generated in the child, which is felt as difficult to understand or accept. He may thus begin to be rendered weak, insecure, and shaky. This can easily be the focal point around which the origin of his difficulties, with increasing frustrations and disappointments, begin to be felt.

What Are Some Reasons for a Child Not Receiving Adequate Resources in His Early Development?

The reasons why a child does not receive adequate love and warmth at this stage of development may lie in the parents' incapacity to convey it, because of their own problems. This may be expressed either openly in the form of hostility toward an unwanted child; in a detached, disinterested, and aloof parent; or camouflaged in the form of an oversolicitude or the self-sacrificing attitude of an "ideal" mother.

Is Stuttering Primarily a Psychological Problem?

In my opinion, stuttering is definitely a psychological entity. It is an expression of anxiety which arises in a young child who is in conflict, and rendered basically helpless in emotionally insecure and afraid from early childhood. As this kind of a child struggles to combat his inner conflicts, he has too little resources or awareness of what to do or where to turn, in order to release himself from his ambivalent feelings toward his parents and from his emotional entanglements. He feels imprisoned by his own problems and as he makes spasmodic attempts toward some form of integration, he becomes even more frustrated, anxious, and panic-stricken. A vicious circle is created, with too little peace or visible restoration.

In our particular culture, language is considered the chief medium of communication. Through it we express our opinions, feelings, attitudes, and actions. The earliest conflicts of a child are expressed in his communications, both socially and verbally, to his parents and to the outside world about him. Where other children can pass through the primary stages of communication and early development less afflicted, the stutterer, because of his emotionally crippled position, is much more prone to anxiety.

What Are Some of the Possible Psychological Sources That Lead to Stuttering in the Young Child?

The child who tends toward developing stuttering, stems from the following possible sources:

1) Disturbed parental and environmental factors, at an

early age, cause him to become emotionally weakened, and to generate feelings of anxiety with its
accompanying feelings of helplessness and hostility;

2) As a result of the early age at which these threatening sources begin, the child, because of his precarious condition, is unable to organize enough
forces together to restore order to his disorganized
state;

3) As a form of safety and protection to his already
crippled personality, neurotic attitudes are developed,
which because of their compulsive and contradictory
nature, create further conflicts.

4) Since language is the chief medium of communication at this time, it is also the area which first tends
to disorganize when the child's protective structures
are threatened, and as a result give rise to anxiety;

5) The speaking situation, which is normally used to
convey an idea, express a feeling, or ask a question,
now becomes converted into a self-assertive, self-
conscious act in an environment of hostility and fear.
Simple social situations in which speech is required,
unconsciously become oral testing grounds. The
hesitation that results from the conflict between the
rational impulse to speak and the irrational fear of
speaking becomes crystallized as stuttering.

6) At first, the child, except for the expression of some
subjective feelings of tension, awkwardness, or slight
muscular incoordination, is unaware of the serious-
ness of his stuttering condition. However, the added
stresses, fears, threats, and apprehensions of his
anxious parents tend to make the child fix his attention even more on the speaking situation. The
child is now made to feel that when he speaks he
is not perfect, that he is different from others, and
somewhat of a weird creature in society. As a re-

sult, he begins to feel inferior to other children, peculiar and self-conscious.

7) Finally, when this same child enters school, the added stress and the particular competitive atmosphere of this environment further cripple his personality. Speech which is ordinarily not conscious now becomes conscious and identified with fears of both social rejection and the fear of stuttering. The child now becomes and is labeled a confirmed stutterer.

When and How Does Stuttering Begin?

The average age at which children usually begin to stutter is about three years, rarely after the age of nine.

The onset of stuttering in childhood may be precipitated by any experience which is an emotionally inadequate child generates anxiety and fear. Such traumatic experiences may be fright, accident, illness, operations, forcible conversion from left- to right-handedness, or a tense and worrisome home environment. The element of fright as a situational traumatic experience plays the most prevalent role. The most common experiences of this type are: being frightened by the dark or lightning; receiving a severe punishment at the hands of a domineering and stern parent; being frightened by a dog or some other animal; being chased or mobbed by a gang of "tough boys;" being yelled at by an angered person; being thrown unexpectedly into the water for the first time; and being caught in the act of masturbation by a forbidding parent.

The following seven examples are illustrations of some cases of adult stuttering individuals whom I've studied, with known precipitating factors beginning in early childhood:

---

*Case illustrations taken from my book, *Stuttering: A Psychodynamic Approach to Its Understanding and Treatment,* Julian Press, N. Y., 1954.

Case 1

L. H., an only child, was closely attached to his mother, who overprotected him and held him very close to her "apron strings." During his early childhood, she directed his mode of living and shook his feelings of security. She constantly spoke to him of the dangers and cruelties of the outside world, and forbade him to associate with the rest of the boys in the neighborhood. He presented a history of nail-biting, enuresis at the age of nine, and frequent nightmares of a terrifying nature. At the age of six, after much persuasion, he went along with a group of his playmates to a nearby vacant building which his mother had constantly warned him not to visit, because "it was supposed to be haunted." As he entered the building, one of the older boys decided to play a prank on him by pushing him through a doorway and running away with the rest of the group. This incident of being isolated in a forbidden spot was of a frightening nature, and subsequently he stuttered.

Case 2

N. H., a thirty-five-year-old male, was the product of a domineering, stern, and rigid mother and an alcoholic father who had little time to spend with his children. The family environment was one of constant friction and quarrels. At an early age he was subject to nail-biting, temper tantrums, and nightmares of "being beaten up." His eldest brother was his constant and only companion and the one in whom he confided and whom he respected. At the age of eight, while chasing his brother through the streets while playing, he saw his brother struck by a truck and instantly killed. Involuntarily, following this tremendous psychic shock, he began to stutter.

Case 3

R. B., a fifty-year-old female, was dominated most of her life by a tyrannical and intolerant father who punished her frequently. When she was five, she remembers that her mother suddenly became psychotic and was confined to a mental institution. During her early childhood, she was subject to horrifying nightmares of being chased by weird animals which would awaken her and cause her to have nocturnal crying spells. At the age of seven, she was frightened by a large dog, and subsequently began to stutter.

Case 4

S. R., a twenty-year-old male, was the only child of parents who were drug addicts. The father was a severe stutterer, and frequently, when he became angered, would beat his wife in the presence of his son. The mother later took to alcohol and when the boy first entered school, he was shy, seclusive, and insecure. Whenever he was about to be called upon to speak in class, he would become afraid and break out into a complete sweat. His lips would tremble and he couldn't speak for some time. He had been a chronic nail-biter up to the age of fifteen, and there is a history of being a sleepwalker in earlier years. At the age of seven, he was forced, upon the insistence of his father, to undergo a tonsilectomy. The severe fright and shock sustained during this incident were followed by stuttering.

Case 5

D. S., an eighteen-year-old male, went swimming at the age of eight against his mother's wishes. While attempting to dive, he slipped and struck his skull against a plank, receiving a slight injury to his forehead. He was not unconscious, but temporarily shocked and frightened. This frightening experience, plus the anticipation of being punished by his mother, was alleged to have caused his stuttering.

Case 6

A. D., a thirty-three-year-old male, was left-handed since birth. Both parents were described as being vigorous, intolerant, and demanding. There is a history of a brother and a maternal cousin who stuttered. There was a constant fear of not meeting his parents' demands and of receiving some forms of punishment in consequence. As a child, he wet the bed and had frequent nightmares of "falling off tall buildings or of floating off into space, without being able to come back to earth." At the age of five, he was forcibly threatened to be converted from left- to right-handedness, and subsequently stuttered.

Case 7

T. R., an eighteen-year-old male, began to stutter at the age of nine, following an attack of encephalitis lethargica. His family history denoted a highly neurotic, temperamental, high-strung, and worrisome mother. The father died when the boy was six years old, cause unknown. A maternal aunt stuttered and later became psychotic. During the entire course of illness, the mother remained constantly at his bedside, sobbed, cried, and prayed continually for his recovery. He had been a chronic nail-biter and wet the bed until the age of twelve.

Is the Child's Speech a Family Affair?

To quote from a recent excellent booklet published by the Speech Foundation of America: "The child's speech is a family affair. Family harmony means clear sailing for the child in his speech efforts, but family disruptions rock the boat. To get the child's speech back on an even keel it may be necessary for the family to take a look at itself, not simply at the child's speech stumblings. If a child begins to repeat, to hesitate, or to block in his speaking, to an excessive degree, some extra family work may be in order. What's happened recently that may have caused the change in speech behavior? Is there a new baby in the house? Has one child lost the spotlight of family attention? Can we offset a bit our natural tendency to shower our love and praise on the new arrival? Is it hard for a young child to have the whole pie, then find he must share it."

How Do Family Disruptions Disturb a Child's Ability to Speak Well?

Disruptions in the family setting can be disturbing to a child's emotional security and to the further development of his speech, in the following ways:

1. Tensions in the home leading to rejection of the child by the expression of open resentment, too many sharp words, angry words, or words hastily spoken serve as poor models for the child learning to speak.

2. The child may be caught in a cross-fire of conflicts between the parents concerning his behavior and conduct. He is thus rendered ambivalent, torn and confused by conflicting demands or lack of direction. His speech reflects such conflicts and he becomes as a whole anxious, afraid and lost.

3. A very sudden change in environment may throw a sensitive child off stride. Moving to a new neighborhood is one example: lack of familiarity with surroundings and the necessity of talking with strangers may produce speech shyness or hesitancy.

4. As a result of a sudden disruption brought about by a breaking up of the family, for instance following a marital separation, divorce, or the death of one of the parents, usually the father.

5. Finally, the child may be harassed by an overbearing father, a nagging and perfectionistic mother, or even a possessive mother. There may be a bullying brother, or a domineering and tormenting sister. The home may lack tranquility; there may be too much noise and aimless activity, much running and bustling, much calling from room to room, and a total absence of calm.

In What Manner Does the School Period Influence the Development of Stuttering?

The period spent in school, which every child in our particular culture undergoes, leaves behind it many revealing impressions of growth experiences. The child spends in this specific situation at least eight years of his life, several hours a day on the average. His entrance into school is the first crucial parental break, and he begins to experience some of his first attempts to live apart from a protective environment. He begins to sense the first impact of freedom from his parents and a real effort at achieving independence. He is literally thrown into a new social milieu, filled with communal and group activities. It is here that he starts to feel his way through, by creating new behavioral adjustments, comprising a whole new set of values and attitudes. As he struggles with the new routines, demands, and restrictions of his school environment, he finds that he no longer has his own special and treasured privileges, but that he is now considered only a member of a larger social group. Alongside these new experiences, he has to contend with and face up to competitive group situations not present in his own home. In spite of these new situational stresses, a healthy child can make a more or less satisfactory adjustment to this environment, and find in it many pleasant experiences. An insecure and inadequate child in this same school situation can make an unsatisfactory adjustment and exhibit, as a result of this, unhappiness, resentment, broodiness, day-dreaming, and behavioral disorders of all sorts.

What Role Does the Teacher Play in this Period?

The teacher is the most important person to whom the child relates in the school situation. He usually looks up

to her as the supreme authority, with awe and absolute respect. The average child leans toward his teacher for praise,
admiration, recognition, and approval. In the eyes of most
children, she becomes an omnipotent figure, sometimes
having a greater influence on children than do their parents. Upon her shoulders rests the constant evaluation of
her pupils; and because of this responsibility; she may
easily be unjustly admonished and blamed by many
parents.

What Is the Period of Quickest Development of Speech?

The period of the quickest development of speech is generally considered to occur during the fourth and fifth developmental years of life. It is somewhere in this period
of growth that the child begins to sense being filled with
an overabundance of desires and needs to express himself openly, and that the inhibiting influences of tense and
perfectionistic parents can be significant trauma to the
future function of the particular child's speech mechanism.
Entrance into school following this period can prove quite
difficult.

Why Is the School Setting So Important to the Stuttering Child?

The school setting is generally the one place where a
stuttering child first comes into awareness in terms of the
outside world. Where he may once have first felt that his
environment was a safe and protective one, he now discovers the first real pangs of social disapproval and non-
acceptance. He begins to feel different from his classmates,
finds that he is afflicted with a defect, considers himself
peculiar, and feels basically different, estranged and remote.
As he attempts to struggle and make greater and more
desperate efforts with his speech difficulty, he finds the

results even worse. He becomes all the more frustrated, anxious, angered; he feels trapped, at odds with himself, and generally hopeless. He feels inferior, ashamed, ridiculed, and embarrassed as he considers the question, "Why can't I talk like the others?" He develops an exaggerated social awareness, and there is the beginning of the emphasis on his speech as a conscious, deliberate and controlling process. In school, he usually restrains himself from being involved in any situation which is competitive or which may necessitate the use of talking. He generally sits in the rear of the class, rarely initiates discussion or answers questions spontaneously; and he avoids most situations which might provoke the slightest fear of stuttering. Even though he may be intellectually superior to most of his classmates, he minimizes his own potentialities, capacities, and gifts by remaining silent and not risking the possibility of a stuttering effect. Sight or hearing difficulties, at this time which are not corrected may further aggravate his speech condition. These physical defects are often overlooked, either through a lack of awareness on the part of the teacher, the refusal of proud parents to accept the existence of these conditions, or the unwillingness of the child himself to admit his incapacities through fear of parental punishment.

Is the Stuttering Child a Sensitive Individual?

The stuttering child is a hypersensitive and "touchy" individual. He reacts keenly and strongly to any environmental pressures, coercion, or criticisms from others, joking of the other children, or even the slightest degree of disciplining. Because of the stuttering child's special delicate subjective responses, his presence in the classroom, for instance, is generally felt acutely by his classmates and teachers. His slow, awkward, and hesitating speech usually make him the butt and victim of many of the children's jokes and pranks. His position adds to the teacher's everyday classroom difficulties. She is in a most precarious situation, for if she approaches the stuttering child with an attitude of pity and compassion, she then is faced with the question of rendering him special privileges—thus setting in motion a basis for using them for future claims. If she ignores his condition, this reaction may add all the more to his feelings of rejection and hurt. Should she bring into play her own anger and hostile feelings, she not only engenders further fear and withdrawal in this sort of child, but has also to contend with reprisals and vindictiveness from his parents. Only through a real understanding, with consistency and a constructive feeling for these particular children, can the classroom teacher properly handle the problem.

Chapter 3

THE STUTTERING PROCESS

How Does a Person Who Stutters Differ Basically from Other Neurotics?

The person who tends toward stuttering, though basically similar in personality to other neurotics, may be said nevertheless to present characteristic differences in his orientation toward life.

To begin with, the stutterer feels at most times apart and different from others in his society. He feels that although others also have difficulties in life, they can cope with them and live much more easily with their problems. He feels more permanently crippled than others because of the fact that he cannot hide or conceal his speech difficulty. Therefore, he is the constant target of their embarrassment, ridicule, and disapproval. He may rationalize to the effect that persons with migraine headaches, asthma, stomach ulcers, etc., suffer, but they can still keep their troubles to themselves and go on living, while he being unable to speak fluently, has the added burden of social criticism and judgment. As a result, he may feel that the world should provide him special services and privileges and entitle him to a "position in life," "a job suitable to his speech incapacity," "a society which will make allowances for his stuttering," yet at the same time not make it appear too obvious that he is crippled. Along with these notions, he may feel embittered and blame his particular culture, with its telephones, dictaphones, and other means of verbal communication.

What Irrational Demands Does the Stutterer Make Upon Others?

Since he most times feels ostracized and a "victim of his society," the stutterer tends to demand that certain "special privileges and rights" are due him. Others should take over for him in those verbal situations where he might encounter some difficulty. They should answer the telephone for him, make requests for him, give him exact information, and pay him absolute attention whenever he talks. He feels that these are his due since he then "does not have to go through the bother and inconvenience of repeating himself and thus stuttering all the more." The reasoning here is, "that since you know that I stutter in these particular situations, you should understand me perfectly well the first time and help me to avoid further embarrassment and ridicule."

What Specifically Does the Stutterer Demand of His Listeners When He Speaks?

When he begins to speak, he may feel entitled to absolute attention and the fullest of interest on the part of his listeners. Since he stutters, he feels that he has to weigh carefully his words before talking, and as a result what he says is of the utmost value. People should be considerate and not interrupt him when he is speaking. They should never restrict him into giving exact responses or concrete facts when conversing with him. People should not ask him directly such exacting questions as: "What is your name and address?" "How can I get to such and such an address?"

As he speaks, others should not look away, yawn, or appear in any way distracted. When they call him by telephone, they should realize that he stutters, speak to him softly, and not become annoyed or harsh should he have difficulty. He should never be called on to testify in court, read in class, make reports to a group, or be held to specific reading situations. Little does he know, or want to know, that many other people also have difficulties when speaking, but his rationalization here is that "Yes, but they don't stutter!"

How Does a Stutterer Usually React in Competitive Situations?

In competitive situations, though basically aggressive, the stutterer most times feels inclined to lean over backwards and demand that others take the initiative. Again, since he stutters, he expects others to make things easy for him, especially in the speaking situation. Since pressures cause him to stutter, he expects others to understand his sensitive position and place few obstacles or difficulties in his path. Though he may be harsh and critical of others' shortcomings, he feels that he in turn should be understood and respected at all times. When he stutters, he magically wishes and demands others to ease his dilemma, yet not to expose the fact that he is having difficulty in speaking. Others should substitute for him in trying competitive spots, do the detailed work for him, take over for him when he has to talk—yet not rob him of the prestige and glory which he feels is coming to him. His rationalization here is: "I know I can do the work much better than most people. My only problem is that I stutter when I have to express myself. Therefore, since I was born to stutter, and can't help myself, I'm entitled to at least the praise for my hidden talent and abilities. Others should recognize the 'truth'—that if I didn't stutter, how simply I would be able to master many of these same situations."

Does the Stutterer Hide Behind His Stuttering in Job Situations?

In job situations, he usually blinds himself to the reality that he avoids not only situations where he may have to speak, but many others. When this is brought to his attention, he may be compelled to agree to this fact, but then quickly turns about and feels that situations in which he must talk do not enter into the picture and are of minor importance. In competitive areas, he shirks responsibilities and avoids most struggles, yet basically gripes and complains that he never gets a "fair break." Because he fears talking, he narrows his activities and duties to a minimum. He feels for the most part ignored, apart from his working colleagues, and harbors many times the attitude that he is being exploited and abused.

How Does the Average Stutterer Respond to Coercion?

The person who tends toward stuttering is generally adverse to any form of coercion, implicit or explicit. In relation to others, he feels he should not have to be held to specific rules or regulations, regardless of their validity. He usually rebels against such rules, becomes indignant, and feels them as an imposition upon his privacy. He *should not* have to be at work at a specific time, regulate his time to bus or train schedules, or be subjected to questioning or examination. In situations where he cannot rebel or avoid feeling coerced, he retaliates by unconsciously protesting with the use of his stuttering.

What Magical Expectations Does the Stutterer Make Upon Women in General?

A stutterer will be attracted to a female partner who may impress him as being stronger or superior to others, thus serving as an unconscious protection against his own weakened and threatened ego. For, he rationalizes, that if he can depend upon his choice of partner for protection and safety, then he can become invulnerable to the many hurts and frustrations he experiences as coming from the hostile world about him.

He magically expects this partner to surrender herself totally to all his whims and needs as they arise. She should foresee any difficulties he may have, especially in the speaking situation. She should cover up for his stuttering, talk for him whenever she senses he might begin to stutter, without exposing his impediment or embarrassing him in the presence of others. Not only should she be able to meet these emergencies, but she should be able to do so with poise and grace, without making him appear weakened or foolish. She should magically move in and out of these difficult speaking spots without being too obvious about it, and always be sufficiently keen and alert not to assume too much the center of the stage. She should then withdraw at an opportune moment, allowing him to re-enter nonchalantly and resume his role in the group with eclat and a semblance of strength.

Even though he may consider his partner the superior and stronger one, the stutterer secretly believes himself to be the master and "real magician."

His partner should magically turn on and off her emotions to suit his particular moods. She should guess, without his communicating to her, those moments in which he may feel lonely, saddened, hurt, or even conflicted. At these times, he may demand from her all sorts of reactions, ranging from understanding, sympathy, closeness, and warmth to wanting to be left alone in utter privacy. At still other times, there may be a complete switch of his own feelings to gladness, joy, elation, or even hilarity; he will expect her to feel similarly and react accordingly, no matter what her own personal feelings or reactions may be at the time.

How Does the Stutterer React to Others in the Speaking Situation?

He usually appears self-effacing and in constant dread of

appearing superior to others in verbal situations. He may speak only when asked to, or when questioned directly. On his own, he may have an idea to contribute something which he feels strongly about, but then either squelches it or denies its expression in the open. He may rationalize this action of his on the grounds that what he was about to say wasn't important enough to begin with, or that "since he stutters" he'd better not talk about it unless it be absolutely imperative to do so. At other times, he may lean over backwards or cringe with fear at the thought of exercising an assertion or expressing a conviction. He feels at these times inferior to others, and thinks that others despise him and accuse him, not for himself necessarily, but again because "he is a stutterer." He feels others don't have the time or patience to listen to or wait for him as he undergoes the torture of "pushing out his words." He further feels others don't realize how much he suffers and struggles at these times and that "fate has been cruel to him in rendering him a cripple for life." In these self-recriminatory phases, his voice becomes small, weak, hardly perceptible, and hesitations between words become all the more prolonged. In these intense struggles where he has to mobilize every possible energy to keep going, he feels simultaneously an inner feeling of failure and doom. His previous convictions or assertions become lost in the shuffle, and what he now expresses in its place are increased tension, vagueness, and profuse apologies. He feels rendered helpless, confused, torn, anxious, and all the more hopeless about himself. It isn't too difficult to understand the intense amount of suffering and misery which such a person experiences in these particular conflicting situations.

How Do these Self-effacing Attitudes Reinforce the Process of Stuttering?

The stutterer is, because of emotional make-up, in constant dread of failing in the speaking situation. Before he even begins to speak, he is generally overwhelmed with the fear of not being able to initiate the utterance of a single sound or word. In situations where he feels threatened, he whips up and distorts the facts of the actualities, to a state of feeling it to be a calamity or doomed to fail. He now feels, "I won't be able to even open my mouth," "I can't do it, I'm sure I'll stutter badly," or, "It will be so bad that I'll probably stop speaking somewhere in the middle and be paralyzed with panic," etc. He fears this intense ridicule, criticism and embarrassment; not as his own self-recrimi- nations, but as coming somewhere from the outside and from others. Since he is driven compulsively toward the achievement of perfection in speaking, his main emphasis is directed not in terms of what he wants to express, but how he will "say it," and what sort of impression will he make before others when he speaks. His profound sense of inadequacy and worthlessness in the speaking situation compels him to experience each new attempt at speaking as a testing ground for his actual existence.

Do Some Stutterers Tend to Minimize Their Stuttering?

Some stutterers use expansive attitudes to cover up their shortcomings. Instead of dreading their affliction, they brag about the definite advantages they, as stutterers, have over average speakers. Some of them take great pride in identi- fying themselves with stutterers who have accomplished great things in spite of their speech difficulty, such as Sir Winston Churchill or Somerset Maugham. Gottlober de- scribes this rather well when he says: "In a more serious vein, a number of blockers have expressed the feeling that there was a certain distinction in having a speech deviation. It set them off from the mob. In a sense, they were 'a chosen people.' They stood out with a select few in a way which had more advantages than the uninitiated could know about. They felt they were quickly singled out in a group, and once met were seldom forgotten. Another thought often expressed is that only intelligent people block; 'it takes brains.' (Many laymen have the opposite impression.) Some claim halting and repetitious speech is typical of those who are deep thinkers. To support this delusion, we have known a number of normal speakers who simulated a mild form of blocking because they too thought it was indicative of profound thinking, or, more often, simply because they were trying to attract attention. Another instance in which blocking has been considered a mark of distinction is related in a story about a prince of long ago who was a severe blocker. So proud was he of his halting speech that he issued a degree stating that blocking was a royal prerogative, and anyone not of princely blood who spoke in similar fashion would meet death by the axe."

What Would Be an Example of an Expansive Stutterer?

One patient of mine who stuttered very badly first entered into treatment assumedly because of other problems, making no mention at all of his difficulty in speaking. It was not until three months later that I brought up this issue of his stuttering. He then became quite indignant, blushed profusely, and made every attempt to deny the existence of any speech difficulty. What he felt was that there was really nothing markedly wrong with his speech, but that when he became excited he only had such difficulties as any other person might have. This person was an extremely expansive individual, who in his own evaluation of himself attempted to deny any imperfection in his personality. It was not only his speech difficulty that he refused to admit to himself, but many other defects, which at first sight did not enter into the realm of stuttering. He drove himself desperately, for instance, into trying to prove that he could accept jobs and obligations pertaining especially to the speaking situation. Though he possessed special abilities in writing, he still felt that in order to be a "good writer" one should be able to also be an "excellent lecturer." In other words, he rationalized to himself: "In order to write well, I should be able to speak well." Eventually, his repeated difficulties in the speaking situation led him to depreciate his writing as well, and finally the validity of the ideas which he sought to express. I tried to help him understand that he would have to realize his own limitations; although he could and did write well, it was not feasible to expect comparable proficiency in speaking. He still resisted and fought me, and refused quite tenaciously to admit to his stuttering. This example will illustrate in what ways a person who stutters may add to his dilemma by the impossible demands which he makes upon himself. For, even though a person may stutter, he can still express his capacities and potentialities in our culture without the absolute necessity of being an eloquent and perfect speaker.

How Does a Stutterer Exhibit Attitudes of Resignation?

The person who stutters can restrict his wishes in many spheres of life, including that of verbal communication. The very intent to speak becomes objectionable to him, and implied in its make-up are many self-imposed prohibitions. He feels very little choice of words, and since he resents being trapped, coerced, and pushed into talking, his escape lies in withdrawal or avoidance. He restricts his thoughts and comments to a minimum, speaking only when he feels it to be essential. In this process of resignation, he keeps in check many of his true inner feelings and convictions.

In the actual verbal encounter, the stutterer uses various

methods of detaching and withdrawing himself. At the first indication of difficulty, he draws back immediately from the "painful situation" and refuses to make any real efforts or struggle toward recapturing stability. He may stop in the middle of a sentence, shrug his shoulders with an attitude of "I don't care," or assume a smile of indifference. Any attempt to help him through these embarrassing episodes is met with irritability, annoyance, or even rage. To show real concern for his suffering in these situations, or to encourage him to continue once he is over the initial anxiety, is of little avail. A characteristic retort is: "It can't be so important that you would want me to repeat it." Or, in more vindictive moods, the response may be much stronger.

What Are Some Examples of Resignation in Stuttering?

One stutterer, in one instance in therapy, felt so hopeless and resigned about his speech impediment that for days at a time he carried on most of his conversation by writing his communications on a pad. He used vocal expression only when absolutely necessary, or when he felt comfortably certain of not having any difficulties or inconveniences in the speaking situation. Another developed his own technique of speaking in monosyllabic speech so that he could control his voice when conversing with others. His reasoning was that if he spoke slowly, softly, quietly, and without undue stress or excitement, the probability of his stuttering would be lessened. What he failed to see, of course, was that such an attitude regarding his verbal expressions resulted in his having to suppress much of the real enthusiasm and aliveness that goes with healthy verbalization.

Many other stutterers have been known to withdraw physically from others into an isolated, inconspicuous existence. There are instances of those who have never married, who avoid social contact of most kinds, and who live very much like hermits. Others even go to the extreme of avoiding buses, restaurants, or other public places where they might have to express themselves verbally in order to communicate with others. These and many other desperate maneuvers indicate the extremes to which stutterers may be driven so that they can avoid feeling conflict of any sort, especially in the speaking situation.

How Does the Stutterer Tend to Compensate for His Inferiority in Speaking?

The stutterer attempts to compensate for his inferiority by creating a false image of himself with which he attempts to restore psychic unity, and to rise above his own conflicts. Being divided within himself renders him weakened and with a feeling of unrelatedness. The creation of a false image of himself temporarily gives him a feeling of identity, control, and significance. In this process of self-idealization, which I refer to as the *Demosthenes Complex*, the stutterer goes up into his imagination where he can compensate for his feelings of inadequacy by endowing himself with illusory powers and exalted notions of himself.

In the attempts to achieve these imaginative heights, the stutterer has a complete disregard for feasibility. He knows he has stuttered for years. He also knows that he finds it extremely difficult to speak in certain situations. Nevertheless, he magically feels that someday, without effort or much struggle, his stutter will leave him and he "will become a perfect speaker." When he speaks, he carries the secret and fantastic notion that "this next time he will not stutter." Even as he speaks, he magically hopes to keep out of others' awareness the fact that he stutters. He will resort to forced hesitations, bugaboo words, various bodily meneuvers, twitches and contortions, to distract his audience from becoming aware of the obvious fact that he is stutter-ing. When he begins to speak, should he feel threatened, he demands of himself that he should not be tense or anxious. On the contrary, he should be utterly calm and controlled. He should speak spontaneously at all times. Never be afraid. Never falter. Never grope for a word. He should be "smart," witty, clever—"the center of at-traction."

Does the Stutterer Feel at Times That He Can Consciously Control His Stutter?

He does feel that he should be able to "conquer" his stuttering by sheer conscious control. He feels he should be omnipotent enough "to master it" with the slightest of effort. Operating in this context is another "should" that remains largely unconscious. This "should" demand of him that he be able to turn his stuttering off whenever it suits him. For example, when he feels helpless and a need to cling, he should be able to (and does) exploit his stuttering for all its worth and without compunction. But when he wants to shine, to command, to convince, he should be able by calling on his will power to speak fluently and impressively and not stutter at all.

How Does the Stutterer Tend to Cope with Problems Which Become Unbearable?

When he feels his problems as unbearable, the stutterer usually resorts to projection. He now imposes the re-sponsibility for his conflicts upon others and on to the outside. He will now feel that "others cause him to stutter," or "others expect too much of him when he speaks and he, therefore, becomes rattled and unnerved and stutters." He may feel that he is being coerced into saying exactly what others expect of him, since most people are aware of his stuttering and, therefore, take advantage of his weakness. As a result he is rendered helpless when pushed and becomes inwardly anxious and pressured to the extent that he stutters compulsively. What he fails to understand here is that these are for the most part his own inner demands and expectations of wanting to anticipate and measure up to everyone else's desires and that in reality he is his own worst enemy.

What Are the Consequences of Self-criticism in Stuttering?

These consequences are varied and usually of a destructive nature. The first is in the compulsive need for people who stutter to constantly compare themselves with practically everyone with whom they come into contact. They place themselves at a disadvantage by feeling that the other person is usually the better speaker, more intelligent, better-looking, more interesting, more influential, etc. These comparisons are predominantly so in the speaking situation where the stutterer constantly compares himself to those about him. What he fails to see at these times, however, is that in these comparisons he really does himself an injustice. This is so because he compulsively chooses people with a superior talking ability with whom to compare himself. For example, he will destructively choose to compare himself with experienced and eloquent speakers. As he sits there quietly listening, he beats himself and becomes filled with anxiety and apprehension when he discovers that he, himself, is nowhere near this stage of development. He will belittle himself and feel that he is a "total failure in life," because others speak much better than he. In some instance, this process of self-criticism will cause him to withdraw himself from others, increasing all the more his obsession of himself as a victim of society. As a result of all this, he may become further resigned and hopeless as his stutter worsens.

Does the Process of Stuttering Lead to Inner Psychic Division?

In the process of stuttering, as in any other neurotic process, the individual finds himself divided within himself. He is possessed by many conflicting tendencies which rob him of experiencing himself as a whole. At these times, he has little feeling of his own body. He may appear to be hazy, confused, and his body sensations may be numbed. In the speaking situation, his own voice may be alien to him. When he speaks, he does not feel and experience his own voice as coming from within himself, and being his, but as coming from somewhere outside. Before he starts to speak, a glazed expression covers his face. He finds it extremely difficult to answer questions and comment on remarks addressed to him. He looks through people, rather than at them; a kind of mental paralysis and terror sets in at the mere idea of speaking before a group. He does not feel as though he is actually doing the speaking, but of the speaking situation as being the more compelling and active force. He does not feel as though "I shall speak, I am speaking, or I will speak," but in terms of "I should speak, I must speak, and I have to speak."

Does the Stutterer Depend Solely upon the Spoken Word for Communication and Self-expression?

The stutterer depends mainly upon the spoken word for communication and self-expression. His exaggerated sense of responsibility for speaking robs him of spontaneity, flexibility, and a feeling for inner choice when expressing himself. Some stutterers are known to assume certain roles when speaking and change to others at different times with little feeling awareness. For instance, we know of those who can speak well in their capacities as teachers or administrators, yet stutter badly in other speaking situations. A change in social status can throw a stutterer's equilibrium off balance, and cause him to feel further threatened and chaotic.

How Does the Stutterer Usually Picture Himself in His Own Imagination?

In his own fantasies and daydreams of himself, he usually pictures himself as a great orator. A patient of mine who stuttered badly took great pride in recording his own voice on a wire recorder. He would shut himself in his room, lower the shades, close his eyes, and become filled with an exhilarated feeling of omnipotence as he pictured himself as Abraham Lincoln reading the Gettysburg Address. He would speak in a slow and deliberate manner, using the proper pauses and enunciation, and rarely ever stuttering. When he played back the recording, however, he became overwhelmed with fear and panic. His heart would pound forcibly, his hands would sweat, and he could not recognize the voice which he now heard as being his own. He was highly secretive concerning this recording of his, kept it locked away in his closet, and felt that the very touch of it conveyed a mystical influence. At those times when he felt, as he put it, "stupid or like a dope," he would get, in spite of the accompanying anxiety, a sensation of reassurance and restoration in listening to this recording of his voice.

What Is another Example of Self-idealization in Stuttering?

Another individual I knew who stuttered would prepare himself for the "inevitable," before meeting with a group, by memorizing accounts of special events, data, and "knock-em-dead" remarks, as he called them, so that he would not appear dull and stupid. He felt he had to continually outsmart others, not only with facts, but in the way he could use these facts when he spoke. In these secretive preparations of his, he would pace up and down his room, gesticulate with his hands, and attempt to speak with utter calm and control. Here again, as in the first example, he experienced a great deal of anxiety, but rarely stuttered. Yet, in the actual group situation, this same person, once he found himself caught in contradictions, stuttered badly. He would then feel beaten, frustrated, and basically hopeless. Experiences of this sort, however, did not tend to cause him to take stock of himself, for compulsively he would be driven to perfect himself all the more the next time. Still another person I worked with in psychotherapy, refused to admit in reality that he stuttered too much or that it bothered him too greatly when he spoke. For years, he directed most of his energies and resources toward denying any awareness of imperfection in himself by moving up into his imagination where he would become a "master of the spoken word." He was compulsively driven to seek jobs where the use of an ability to speak was of prime importance. As a result he failed successively as a salesman, a store clerk, and as a law student. Had he faced his stuttering more realistically, he would have chosen field of endeavor where speaking is not of prime importance, and made a success of his efforts.

Is the Symptom of Stuttering Used at Times as a Means of Expressing Repressed Anger?

Stuttering is used by some stutterers as a tool of hostility. With his stuttering, he can make others feel uncomfortable in his presence. He can attempt to intimidate those who easily become guilty and embarrassed by the feeling that they may in some way be to blame for his stuttering. He can arouse anger and hostility in the more aggressive person, and push away or involve those who avoid meeting with him once he begins to stutter. So that, although stuttering may bring an individual a degree of conflict and suffering, it also has at times a secretive and prideful meaning, enabling such a person to restore his weakened ego when he feels frustrated or in a threatened emotional position.

Is Much Psychic Energy Used Up in the Process of Stuttering?

The individual who stutters, like any other neurotic, lives with many unresolved conflicts. As a result, there is a devastating waste of energies which are demanded not only by the existing conflicts themselves, but also by the all-around attempts to remove these conflicts. The stutterer, for instance, is forever worrying about his stuttering. A great deal of his energies go into this process. He also uses a great deal of his energies in the conflicting and contradictory tendencies which are constantly being experienced by him. In the verbal situation, much energy is being used up and misdirected in the overwhelming anxieties and apprehensions associated with the actual speaking itself. Much energy is also used up in the wavering and procrastinating which the stutterer is constantly involved with. He fears taking responsibility for many situations including that of his own speech. He is constantly plagued with the thoughts, and doubts, as to when to talk, should he wait to express himself later, will he stutter, etc.? He is in constant struggle with himself and the world about him. With his continual verbal maneuvering, evasions and bugaboos, he is unable to discover what he really feels or intends to express. All of those compulsions take much energy away from his "real self," and leave the stutterer for the most part inert, resigned, and at times hopeless about his problem.

How Does a Stutterer React When He Is Through Speaking?

When he is through speaking and has had a bad time of it, he usually finds himself lost, shaking, and fumbling blindly to restore his psychic equilibrium. His environment now appears strange and new to him. He feels helpless, embarrassed, need support, and as he tries to get hold of himself, his immediate remarks usually are "What have I said? Was it clear? Did I have much trouble speaking? Did I stutter badly?" At the same time he fears and resents any reference to his stuttering, and detests any kind of criticism, no matter how constructive it may be. He cares little whether he has contributed anything when he speaks, or whether he was interesting or stimulating. His speech, to the exclusion of everything else, is his greatest concern and worry. His egocentricity causes him to resort to the same persistent questions: "How perfectly did I speak? Were others impressed? Did I stutter?"

Is the Stutterer Threatened by the Sound of His Own Voice?

The very sounds and words he utters become both threatening and frightening to him, many times to a near state of panic. When this occurs, oftentimes he may not even be able to identify with his own body, far less hear himself speak. He feels trapped, cornered, and then the race begins: Hurry! Get it over with! Let the beginning be the end! Finish before the stuttering gets too bad! When he finally is through speaking, he feels frustrated, defeated and beaten. He is torn between remaining in the situation and returning to his listeners for some understanding and sympathy; yet his pride interferes, for experiences of this sort he feels as being humiliating and embarrassing. He wants to return and magically straighten out what he believes had previously happened when he spoke, but when he cannot realistically do so, he then finds himself in further conflict. Should he remain and place himself at the mercy of his audience, or should he run and lose face? Both of these extremes are unbearable and offer no practical solution.

Is There an Optimistic Side to Stuttering?

There certainly is! Once the stutterer can take responsibility and face his dilemma squarely, with or without his stuttering, then can he hope for some therapeutic cure and a life of enjoyment and productive existence. At this time, he will regard himself more as a human being, become less involved in his stuttering per se, and will tend to use his energies toward living realistically and not toward self-destruction.

Chapter 4

STUTTERING AS A DISORDER IN COMMUNICATION

How Does Stuttering Relate to the Process of Communication?

Stuttering tells us that communication as a whole, and not just verbal communication, is impaired if it has not actually broken down. In the child, stuttering tells us that emotional communication, in the sense of emotional rapport and give-and-take, wholesome harmony as well as wholesome friction, has been impaired and has perhaps even broken down between the child and one or both of the parents. A happy change in the emotional climate at this time can help matters. If, on the other hand, communication breaks down at this early age, then the process worsens and spreads throughout life to include siblings, parent-surrogates, teachers, authority figures, and finally most everybody indiscriminately becomes a threat and serves as a trigger factor to set off the stuttering. The stuttering then becomes more and more compulsive.

What Is Meant by Language Behavior?

In order to arrive at a deeper understanding of the total personality structure of the person who stutters, we must of necessity gain some insight into his "language behavior." As he speaks, and especially when he stutters, it is imperative that we attempt to penetrate his inner defenses, and decipher some of the stutterer's hidden feelings and thoughts. If we go behind the scenes, especially at the time of his heightened anxiety and stuttering, we shall be able to unravel some of the confusions and hidden implications and mysteries implicit in his stuttering. Finally, we can make an attempt, especially as therapists, to understand not only his objected or external speech, but his subjective, hidden or internalized speech as well.

Is a Knowledge of Symbolic Language of Importance in Understanding Stuttering?

I feel it is basically essential that if we are to clarify the complexities of stuttering, that we have some knowledge of the stutterer's symbolic language. By symbolic language is meant the experiencing of inner feelings, moods, wishes or thoughts, as if they were actualities in the outer world. An example of symbolic deciphering is the attempting to grasp the full meaning behind such a simple expression from a stutterer as: "I'm stuck with a word, I can't go on talking." At face value, it is meant to express just what it verbally states. That is, the specific individual is having difficulty speaking and can't seem to get past a particular "feared" or "bugaboo" word. However, once we go behind the hidden implications we can arrive at a much deeper understanding of his state of chaos and disorganization. What he now seems to be conveying to us in symbolic fashion is that he inwardly feels anxious and helpless in the face of overwhelming threats to his psychic structure. He is also revealing, that being "temporarily stuck with a word or two," threatens his image of himself as the "perfect and lucid speaker," and that as a result he will meet with disapproval from his listeners. As a result of his inner dilemma, the stutterer now feels unable to struggle with his problem and projects all of it to the outside—that which is now expressed overtly is known as stuttering. The stutterer, once he blocks, feels this blocking and inhibition with his whole personality—resulting in final disturbance of feelings, thinking, and actions.

How Does the Speaking Situation Manifest Itself in the Stuttering Process?

The onset of verbal communication begins early in life. The child at this period of development discovers that he is able to express through words and gestures his inward wants and desires. He also discovers that he is not a totally independent being, but dependent upon his environment for acceptance and social approval. He further discovers that his earliest conflicts become expressed in his communications, both verbally and social, in relation to his parents. Where serious conflicts arise, the protective structure of a child's personality become threatened, anxiety is generated, and it is in the specific area of verbal communication that it is first experienced and expressed. Finally, the speaking situation, which is normally used to convey an opinion, an attitude, a feeling, or an assertion, becomes a situation identified and experienced with fear and hostility. The speaking situation now automatically becomes a conscious act, and the forerunner of future difficulties and uncertainties in such a disturbed child. Each subsequent attempt to speak when under similar conditions is met with further increasing doubt, fear, apprehensions, and anxieties. The hesitation that results and crystallizes into what is later known as stuttering results from the conflict between a rational desire to speak and express one's self and the opposing conflicting situations which arise as a result of speaking.

What Are the Stutterer's Attitudes Toward Himself When Speaking?

The very intention to speak to the stutterer has an objectional significance; the mere thought of speaking carries with it a common denominator of fear, dread and apprehension. He starts with the feeling that speaking is a dangerous area in which he is bound to fail. His personality is set immediately into gear for "imaginary battle," which he perceives as about to begin once he starts to talk. Inwardly he feels anxious, disorganized, confused. These diffuse and extreme reactions originate usually even before the utterance of a single word, and are entirely out of proportion to the realities of the situation. Anticipatory reaction of fear and a dread of speaking may be present in any of us before specific speaking situations which are felt as threatening, such as speaking before a group, appearing in court as a witness, etc. However, to the stutterer, almost *any* intent to speak, be it threatening or not, is experienced with marked anxiety and with a diffuse feeling of fright. Since the stutterer has had repetitive experiences of difficulties in speaking since a child, for him the speaking situation continues to be experienced as an automatic threatening situation, no matter what the actualities of the experience itself.

Once the Stutterer Does Begin to Speak Can He Adopt Himself to Depend upon His Own Natural Resources for Spontaneous Verbalization?

Usually not. Instead of depending on his natural resources for speaking, he will resort to various learned maneuvers, evasions, substitutions, and magical rituals. He substitutes an "easy word" for a "feared word," add extraneous words to help him over difficult spots, postpone the utterance of a sound by the use of "ah-ah," or even change the entire context of what he is saying at the time to suit his own devices. Other ways of momentarily releasing anxiety in the speaking situation are by distractions of all sorts, such as pinching himself, talking in a mechanical tone, laughing at a moment of anticipation, looking away, or drawing the listener's attention by some non-speech activity. These releasing devices aid the stutterer to break through a hesitation or block in speaking, but they are basically artificial in nature and actually intensify and engender the stuttering itself.

What Does the Second Stage of Stuttering Involve?

The first components of disturbance and behavior disorganization which occur in the stutterer are basically of an emotional or feeling variety. The second stage in the stuttering process has to do with the many complexities involved in the thought processes preceding the actual verbalization of the spoken word. In this difficult preverbal formative period, the stutterer must contend not only with the actual thought or the meaning of "what he is to say," but many of his energies now become directed into how "should he say it," "when should he say it," also to be able to "say it" without hesitation or difficulty. "He must be able to speak clearly, perfectly, concisely, and in a flawless manner." He must also keep out of awareness stimuli which have caused him difficulty when having spoken in the past. He attempts the latter by keeping the various devices mentioned in smooth operation and under perfect control. Since all of these are in urgent need of attention, and take energy away from any spontaneous verbalization, what results instead is usually confusion, hesitation, and blocking, both of thought and of language. The ultimate result is one of increasing difficulty in speaking, added anxiety, continued dread, further confusion and blocking—thus setting into operation a vicious circle.

How Does the Stutterer Differ from the Average Speaker?

Where the average speaker's attention is proportionate

to his interests in a speaking situation, that of the person who stutters is governed mainly by fear. One usually experiences his speech as his own and as originating from within himself. He feels a choice of his own words or groups of words, though there may be some indecision as to word pronounciation. However, once he decides and voluntarily chooses his words, he will have little difficulty in consummating the speaking itself. The stutterer, on the other hand, generally experiences his speech as foreign to himself and as coming from somewhere outside of himself. As a result of his inner turmoil, he experiences little choice in deciding upon one or another word, but must choose between word *entities*. His dilemma in speaking is experienced not so much in terms of "what to say," but "how to say it."

Does the Stutterer Color a Great Deal of His Speech with His Feelings?

For the most part, he injects a great deal of his speech with the particular mood or feelings he may be experiencing at the time he is speaking. He is unable to keep these varying reactions to himself, but feels compelled and driven to project his feelings when speaking into his speech. Since the success or failure of what he says is highly dependent upon the acceptance or disapproval of others, he gears his speech to meet and suit what he feels as demands coming from others. This accounts for the many fluctuations in mood which are characteristic of people who stutter, and may tend to explain the fact that such people are stutter-free in one particular situation but may stutter severely in another.

Does the Stutterer Usually Demonstrate Rigidity to Change in the Speaking Situation?

Where the average speaker will voluntarily stop speaking

when he anticipates, or is in, difficult speaking circumstances; the stutterer becomes incapable most times of becoming flexible should he begin to hesitate or block. The average speaker is able to interrupt his speech should he feel some disturbance, and resume his speaking at a more suitable level of productivity. The stutterer, however, tends to sabotage his own self-interests when in difficulty in speaking, and activates the unpleasantness of his unfavorable position. The slightest indication of blocking or hesitation before or during the process of speaking disrupts him to an even greater degree of imbalance and chaos. For, to have to admit discrepancies or flaws to his own notion of perfection is a severe blow to his pride. Since he should not have any shortcomings when speaking, and especially since he should remain unruffled when he does demonstrate hesitations in talking, his protective devices become dented and is then experienced as irreparable. He now has to contend not only with an immediate magical restoration of his crumbling superstructure, but is also subject to all the recriminations, embarrassments, and criticisms which he projects to the outside and on to others. At these times, the stutterer becomes further overwhelmed with an attitude of disaster and with a feeling of too little strength or volition on his part of being able to do anything about his precarious position. In these chaotic states, he feels completely and compulsively driven by forces outside himself, at the mercy of his stuttering. He can now only desperately hope to salvage part of himself, and magically wish for some restoration of his ego, yet fear at the same time an impending doom and further stuttering.

What Are the Stutterer's Predominant Attitudes Toward Others When Speaking?

The stutterer is strongly dependent upon the reactions of his audience, be it one or more people. What he fears when speaking depends to some degree on how he may feel he performs in the act itself, and to a large extent also upon the expectant response he anticipates from his listener. Toward others, especially when he speaks, he may experience himself as though he were "on stage." He then sees himself as the performer, at the mercy of his critics— the audience.

Toward others, he is in constant need of their approval, praise, recognition and reassurance. He feels that since he stutters he can make claims upon others for their absolute understanding, sympathy, consideration, and attention. Because of his heightened sensitivity to coercion, criticism, rebuff, or even the slightest denial, his listeners become constant threats to his particular problems; and, the more threatening his audience appears, the greater the amount of rejection will be experienced as forthcoming from others.

Do Many Stutterers Unconsciously Tend Toward Perfection in Speaking?

Many stutterers unconsciously tend toward perfection when speaking. This striving toward self-idealization begins in early childhood, when, with each embarrassing and humiliating experience he received at the hands of others when he stuttered, he vowed to himself that someday he would return and prove to this hostile world about him that he has conquered his impediment and can now speak "perfectly well." Though this attitude, which is filled with feelings of inadequacy, revenge, hostility, triumph and the fear of failure, is intense at the same time it is kept buried, being usually hidden from the stutterer's conscious awareness. What expresses itself in actuality is a conglomeration of conflicting tendencies and feelings which become crystallized and expressed in the form of stuttering.

How Important is the Listener's Response to the Stutterer?

The auditor's response to a stutterer is of utmost significance and it can control to a large extent the stutterer's feeling responses in the speaking situation. The stutterer feels obligated to and tied down by his audience once he begins to speak. He now feels coerced and will attempt to comply entirely with the wishes and demands of his listeners. He struggles, to repeat, not only with "the actuality of verbalizing," but also in what way his listeners will react to him when speaking. While speaking, he is compelled to fix his attention onto his audience, to study their facial expressions intently, and try to decipher every one of his listener's inner thoughts concerning his performance. His own egocentricity demands this attitude in him when he speaks. Since he cannot stand alone on his own self-evaluation and conviction, he arrives at an evaluation of his own status and actions through the opinion and assertion of others. His dire need of winning over his audience, receiving their praise and recognition, drives him further to orientate most of his feelings, thoughts, and actions in terms of meeting the satisfaction of his listeners, and not in relation to his own opinions or wishes. He needs to control his audience and to keep it intact. When he speaks, he demands absolute attention. No one must leave, lest he become irritable, enraged, and so begin to stutter. He feels here that since he makes the sacrifice to give to others when speaking, in spite of his "affliction," others should at least have the decency and patience to sit quietly until he finishes speaking.

Is the Stutterer's Anxiety Usually Ended After He Is Through Speaking?

After he is through with whatever he has to say, he

feels temporarily relieved, but soon after enters into further dismay, confusion, and turmoil. Anxiously, he may now turn to his listeners, to wait with apprehension, for any of their spontaneous remarks concerning his behavior or what he just spoke about. His own conclusion robs him of the possibility of taking stock of his specific role in the speaking situation itself. Though it is quite healthy to want other people's opinions and evaluations of our actions, the stutterer throws the entire weight of his status, especially when speaking, on to his audience. His vanity in imaginatively perceiving himself as a "wonderful and perfect speaker" of necessity compels him to become entirely dependent upon the needs and reactions of the environment about him. Since he feels little of himself at most times, and especially so in the speaking situation, he can come alive only by living vicariously through others.

Does the Process of Stuttering in Itself Drive Other People Away?

The stutterer's detachment, aloofness, callousness, whining, and abused feelings, and not the stuttering itself drive his audience away from him. The stutterer, as much as he stands in awe of other's evaluation of himself, has also a bitter contempt toward them for his having to be so helpless and dependent. Unconsciously, he will exercise his arrogance and use subtle derogatory comments to widen further the gap between himself and his listeners. He in a sense does not talk directly to others, but attacks his listeners either with his stuttering, or when in control of his speech feels as though he is now the stronger in the situation, and can now talk down to his audience. The conflict between the desire to be aloof and utterly independent of others, and the need to feel completely dependent upon his auditors, creates a vicious cycle and ultimately increases his stuttering.

Does the Stutterer Live Through His Own Words?

The stutterer, in a sense, lives through his own words—including both the spoken and the written word. His words have omnipotent significance to him and move along with his image of being "the perfect speaker." His egocentricity compels him to experience objects or things referred to when he speaks as pertaining solely to himself; there is no real audience. Since he feels he has to speak perfectly, he feels in competition with himself and with others. He feels compelled to also use the best descriptive terms, make the most succinct remarks, and have complete understanding or knowledge of whatever he is talking about. To fall short of these expectations in himself makes him feel that he will be rendered vulnerable and a prey to his auditors. To have command over himself at all times in the speaking situation is one of the prime ways in which such a person feels he can protect his weakened structure and gain some form of pseudo-integration.

Does the Stutterer Depend to a Great Extent upon His Words?

He exhibits a great sense of dependence upon his words as the sole means of communication for most of his feelings, opinions and attitudes. He feels that only through words can he make himself understood, and since he feels weak in the speaking situation, his whole approach to communication is distorted. This adherence to words is of a strict and rigid quality. Within himself he feels compelled stringently to use the "perfect word," at the "right time," and "in the right context." He is driven to be perfect, exacting, and absolutely correct in all of his communications.

Does the Stutterer Fear the Omnipotence of Words?

From early childhood, the stutterer is obsessed in believing that the spoken word carries with it an effect of tremendous imprint and impact. The child who stutters, for instance, learns early in life that speaking can upset his whole life and bring about inner chaos and the eruption of fear and anxiety. He also learns through experience that a mastery and control over his words is one of his only means of salvation. He thus finds it imperative to measure his words, to use them with "utter care and caution," and that "a careless word can cause a calamity." The speaking situation becomes his arena of combat—the one place where he can emerge the victor or succumb to the mercy of others.

As the individual continues to grow and develop, he discovers even further the omnipotence of words and thoughts. With words, he finds he can control and master things about him. Using the "right" or the "wrong" word can be of significant importance. "Words can kill and resurrect." "Words are dangerous, powerful, destructive," and should be used with discretion. In people who learn to place an overemphasis on the omnipotent value in words early in life, such as may be found in those who develop stuttering, words become experienced as dangerous weapons. Words become filled with feeling and emotion. They can reveal one's most innermost thoughts, feelings, hostility or vindictiveness. Words, finally, can expose our most impenetrable defenses and readily reveal our truest personality.

What Kind of Behavior Do We Usually Witness in the More Severe Forms of Stuttering?

In the most severe forms of stuttering, one can vividly observe the intense struggle and the presentation of bizarre and grotesque speech behavior patterns. For instance, the stutterer may here begin by discussing a serious matter, suddenly have difficulty in speaking, and anxiously switch

in a phase of many sorts of compulsive, indiscriminate, and disorganized movements. At the point of interruption or hesitation, when the state of anxiety and disruption is usually at its highest level of tension, such an individual may suddenly stop speaking, interrupt his trend of thought; then by some form of magic suddenly begin to whistle, giggle, or smile, splutter, mumble, or give vent to an explosion of words. Some others may, at these periods of chaos, suddenly again break away from the original discussion, start to tell a joke, or even continue by saying something completely out of context with the original idea or premise. In this ritual of unconscious maneuvering is the hidden need of such a person to erase any indication of stuttering to his own awareness and especially from that of his listeners. Little does he know that his hesitations and other manifestations of stuttering might be less obvious and painful to himself and to others than these distorted magic rituals of his which rarely function. In reality, he actually increases the precariousness of his weakened position by engendering additional attention toward his speech impediment.

Only when the stutterer can gain enough inner strength to admit to his shortcomings and give up the use of these magic rituals, will he be able to find real basic balance and ultimately achieve relaxed and spontaneous speech.

Chapter 5

THE PREVENTION AND THERAPY OF STUTTERING

What Can Be Done to Prevent Stuttering?

The Speech Foundation of America encourages the following goals parents should attempt to accomplish in order to ensure speech fluency in the child:

1) Become as sensitive as possible to the infant's many ways of communicating with us—verbally and non-verbally;

2) Tune in more to the *feelings* being expressed, rather than to the fact or intellectual content spoken—*how* one speaks is very often much more crucial than *what* one speaks;

3) Learn what it takes for normal speech to develop— learn the ways of giving a helping hand, and make definite efforts to guide your child's speech development;

4) Provide good models of speaking for your child— you are his first and most important teacher;

5) Learn how to listen, and how not to listen—yes, it takes some doing to know how to listen well;

6) Make your expectations concerning your child's speech and other behavior reasonable—try not to expect too much too soon;

7) Make certain there are plenty of opportunities for feelings to get out into the open—especially the distasteful feelings—not only your child's, but your own as well—then work at figuring out why they built

up and what you can do to improve the situation;

8) Encourage speech spontaneity in your child by strengthening his self-confidence and his desire to share his world with you—as you share yours with him;

9) Be a good conversational partner for your child—too often our conversational traffic-patterns are one-way streets—or dead ends;

10) Keep family relationships as harmonious as possible —especially those between husband and wife for they set the pace and provide the key to successful speech growth.

The very process of reaching, itself, for these goals will improve the possibility of your child's growing up to speak normally.

What Are Some Good Listening Habits Parents Can Develop to Prevent Stuttering in Their Child?

1) Set aside some time each day for each child in your family;

2) Listen with your "heart" and not so much your "head."

3) Don't rationalize or moralize too much, but attempt to listen with an "inner ear of understanding";

4) Be available and responsive when your child speaks;

5) Give your child the fullest of your attention, try not to interfere when he speaks or give the appearance of being bored and disinterested;

6) Draw your child out as he listens; encourage him to want to speak;

7) Try listening not only to the child's words but also to the child himself;

8) Finally, if you can be successful with 50 per cent of the above attempts at reaching the depth of your child, you may consider yourself a good listener.

Is There a Specific Age at Which Treatment of the Stuttering Child Should Begin?

It was once believed that the treatment of stuttering before the age of eight merely tended to fix the stuttering more firmly. It was also felt that treatment in the younger child should be directed solely to the parent, and the child be left alone to grow out of his affliction.

Recent investigations, however, allow us to see beyond this narrow vista and to extend the therapeutic means to the child primarily, and as early as possible, in order to solidify and limit the child's opportunities for normal psychological and speech development.

Can Hypnotism Cure Stuttering?

Though hypnotism and many other brief therapeutic approaches do produce an immediate lessening of the speech difficulty, they accomplish little or nothing in inducing changes in the total personality. A comprehensive therapeutic approach must focus not only on the early conflicts in the child's development, but upon his parental relationships and finally, his attitudes toward himself as a whole. With all of this pertinent data at hand, therapy may then be directed toward a reorientation of the child by making available to him whatever constructive resources are possible toward healthy growth and away from unhealthy emotional development. Once this is accomplished, or is in the process of development, we can expect a gradual lessening of anxiety and an amelioration of the symptom of stuttering itself.

When Should the Actual Therapy of Stuttering Begin?

Since stuttering usually begins at an early age, treatment too should begin as early as possible. For therapeutic purposes we can distinguish two phases of stuttering: primary and secondary. In treatment during the primary stage (five to ten years of age), when the child is less cognizant of and anxious about his speech problem, the approach is mainly one of treating the parents and, through them, removing unfavorable environmental influences. The prime objective is also to treat the child in being able to give support and aiding him to lessen the degree of his inner turmoils and conflicts, to attempt to arrest the disorder, and finally, if possible, to prevent perpetuation of the problem into the secondary stage or into confirmed stuttering.

How Are the Parents Helped During the Early Phases of Therapy?

The parents of the stuttering child are made as aware as possible of the many workable means available to ease the demands made upon their children, and how these same pressures can lead to stuttering. An ideal situation, it goes without saying, would be to encourage both parents to enter into treatment, to help them work through some of their own most disturbing emotional problems, which in turn would better the child-parent relationship. Where this is not feasible or is met with resistance, treatment of parents must assume the form of specific instructions. These instructions are directed toward: (1) improving the general health of the child; (2) the balancing of his environmental tempo, with the removal of some of the more exciting and disturbing tension factors; (3) attempts to encourage in the child a sense of confidence, responsibility, mutual love, and respect; (4) the working toward a sense of coordination and rhythm in the child's personality as a whole; (5) encouragement of the child to feel free to mix spontaneously with other children and especially with members of his own family; (6) to encourage more constructive methods of discipline; (7) to enable the child to grow at his own particular pace and to help him find his own potentialities and creative capacities; (8) to establish a feeling of real love, warmth, and mutual belonging in the family unit; (9) and, finally, to avoid making the child feel unique or different from others, and especially to avoid making him "speech-conscious." In this last context, it is especially urged that the child be allowed a sense of freedom of expression through speech, and a feeling for an independent choice of words.

Why Is it more Desirable to Treat the Stuttering Child as Early as Possible?

In the early years, a child's conflicts are less entrenched and complex than in later years. He has less anxiety to contend with and his neurotic mechanisms are less intricate and closer to the surface of consciousness. The young child also has less of a compulsive attachment to his symptom of stuttering than that of the adolescent or the adult, and he has in his command more constructive forces to do something about it.

What Is the Nature of the Therapy in the Secondary Stage of Stuttering?

In this stage (usually between eleven to nineteen years of age), the stutterer is now consciously aware that he has a speech difficulty and is particularly affected by what others think of him. This adolescent or adult stutterer develops a keen sensitivity around his affliction of speech and his personality in toto assumes specific colorings of anxiety and apprehensions. Treatment in this secondary stage of stuttering, in contrast to that of the primary stage, consists primarily of a direct approach. The individual's problems are tackled directly, and the aim is toward personality reorganization.

Do Many Stutterers Seek Help as a Young Child?

Unfortunately, most stutterers don't come into treatment until they are adults. Many of them, when children, are kept away from treatment through ignorance or "blind spots" in their parents, or else become misled by professionals or so-called authorities who advised that they would "outgrow" the disorder. The tragic result was that they discovered too late that they became, instead, chronic stutterers with a much more serious affliction.

What Are Some Basic Requirements a Therapist Dealing with the Problem of Stuttering Should Have?

The therapist, in order to function at some level of competency, should have most or some of the following essential requirements:

1) He should have an awareness of and an understanding for the person who stutters. Here, having been a stutterer himself will be of obvious benefit. He should also have a reading knowledge of the subject of stuttering, its various theories, its working hypothesis, and its present-day methods of treatment.

2) He should be, in every aspect of his personality, a human being. He should have a feeling for struggle and suffering in humans especially for the person who stutters. In therapy, he should not be aloof or authoritarian, but use constructive assets in himself toward expressing warmth, understanding, sincerity and respect for the patient's own wishes and rights.

3) Be he a psychiatrist, a speech therapist, or a psychologist, he should be well trained in accredited schools or hospitals and clinics. He should also be either certified or an active member in the American Speech and Hearing Association.

4) He should have to some degree a good understanding and be oriented in the dynamics of personality. Along with this knowledge and experience of the human personality, he must have an inherent belief in man's ability to change and grow toward self-realization. He must also have a feeling for process in changing, a knowledge of the patient's fear of it, and the skill to handle defenses against it effectively.

5) Finally, he should have his own problems reasonably well solved, or be sufficiently well aware of them so that they will not interfere with his working constructively with others.

Should the Therapist Make Definite Promises to Parents of a Stuttering Child Concerning the Amelioration of the Symptom?

The therapist should try to help alleviate the parents' anxieties and doubts about their child's future progress by putting them at ease and relating to them in a firm but sincere, warm, open and consistent manner. If the question is made concerning whether the stuttering child can be definitely helped, the answer should not be an immediate and affirmative reply. Instead, the suggestion is made that the therapist might make a remark such as, "Yes, I have no doubts about being able to help your child with his problem, provided there is some real incentive, interest, motivation, and that the job of treatment be a cooperative project." The therapist, instead, who makes rash promises which he does not intend to or cannot fulfill later on, may lead to catastrophic difficulties in the course of treatment. In this same context, the length of time of the individual treatment should be left open and not limited to any definite period.

Briefly What Is Psychotherapy?

Psychotherapy might perhaps best be defined as an effort

at improving the ability of the patient to communicate in a more healthy manner with himself and others. Modern therapy stresses the treatment of the total personality, the whole man, and is directed toward a reorientation of the individual's relations to himself as well as toward his disturbances in relation to others. It also tends to lead the individual out of his unhealthy state by making available to him whatever resources are possible toward healthy growth. The more such a person is helped and directed toward liberating the forces of spontaneous growth, the more awareness, understanding, and sense of being will he have for himself. Hence the ideal in any worthwhile therapeutic approach is the liberation and utilization of those energies and forces which may lead to effective communication and to self-realization.

How Is Psychotherapy Different Today Than in Years Ago?

In the early day, the psychotherapist functioned more as a mirror in which the patient saw his moods, thoughts and feelings reflected. In a conscious effort to maintain himself in a wholly objective fashion and avoiding to involve himself with his patient, the therapist revealed very little of himself as a human being.

Today, the therapist presents himself and communicates with his patient on a more interpersonal basis. He is more involved, and at all times, he strives to communicate with and feel a real interest in his patient, to see him as a suffering entity and to reach within him for what is basically growing and resourceful.

Are the Patient's Words the Most Important in Psychotherapy?

Listening to the words as words only may be most deceiving. In any effective psychotherapy process, the therapist must be keen and alert enough to look behind the patient's contrived screen of verbalizations, nor must he be taken in by the disguising maneuver of this talkativeness. It is essential for him to keep in mind that there is meaning in whatever his patient says, but also in his gestures, movements, facial expressions, tensions, pauses or silences, in his reflections, mannerisms, muscular reactions, and a score of other communing factors.

Is the Language of the Patient in Psychotherapy of Importance?

Only through the sensitive listening to the understanding and recognizing of the secret meanings and the personal character of the language the patient uses—can psychotherapy be successful. When the therapist can receive, record, and decode the patient's verbal and nonverbal impressions successfully, can he assimilate this information, and be able to arrive at an honest evaluation of the problem at hand.

What Information is of Importance to the Therapist in the Initial Interview Concerning the Problem of Stuttering?

The initial interview is a basic source for a number of important facts and data which the therapist must know about his patient before beginning adequate therapy. Briefly, these include: name; age; sex; marital status; occupation; religion; education; social status; family background; sibling relations; medical history; adolescent and adult development; etc. Regarding the specific problem of stuttering the therapist should ask for information pertaining to the age at onset of stuttering, how and where it started, its connection with any traumatic experience or experiences, and when he first began to associate the first objective and subjective feelings of anxiety with his speech defect. In this same context, it is important to seek data concerning the familial history of stuttering, parental attitudes toward his speaking and toward his speech defect, and, most essential of all, the stutterer's own feelings and attitudes about his stuttering throughout his remembered development. Finally, for a more complete picture, it is necessary to have some understanding of his present attitudes about his speech impediment, and especially how he experiences himself with it in relation to himself and others. With all of this data at hand, we can now arrive at a total evaluation of the stuttering problem and the therapeutic approach best suited to fit his needs.

What Basic Essential in the Stutterer Must the Therapist Evaluate Before Planning Any Direct Plan of Approach?

Following the initial interview of one or more sessions, the therapist must evaluate to the best of his judgment and therapeutic acumen the following essential basic criteria:

1) The relative degree of constructive assets and real incentives for help present in the stutterer in relation to opposing negative and retarding forces.

2) The degree and extent of his hopelessness and fear of not being able to ever overcome his speech impediment.

3) The stutterer's extent of awareness of his problems, his real desires for help, the feeling for change, and finally his capacity for cooperation in the therapeutic situation.

4) The degree of severity of his obvious symptoms, and primarily that of his stuttering.

5) Finally, a measure of the stutterer's awareness of and capacity for struggle, a sense for real suffering, and his threshold for anxiety.

Is the Stutterer's Feeling That He is a "Cripple" in our Speech-conscious Society a Difficult Area to Work with?

In people who stutter, there is invested a great deal of

psychic energy invested in the irrational claims they make upon themselves and others. This area presents tremendous resistence to change. To help the stutterer feel that he is not necessarily a "cripple" because he has difficult speech at times, and, therefore, is not entitled to any special privileges from others, is a problem most difficult to tackle. This sort of compulsive behavior comes from two basic sources: from a feeling of being victimized and abused since early childhood, and from the imaginative concept that since "most people have little difficulty speaking and were born with this faculty," that they should be compensated with other privileges.

Which Areas in the Therapy of Stutterer's Provide the Greatest Amount of Difficulty?

1. To encourage the stutterer to being and continue treatment.

Doubts and feelings of doom have become fixed in the minds of those many stutterers who have gone from clinic to clinic, from specialist to specialist, or have been subjected to so-called "miraculous cures." When these same people are initially interviewed for what they may feel is another new and futile attempt, among the many others, they are often skeptical and cautious. At this point, they have little real incentive for receiving help in the solution of their problems, and a difficult area of resistance is set up. The therapist must therefore give a great deal of himself by way of encouragement.

2. To remove those difficulties which are perpetuated by the actual stuttering symptom itself, and the blockage in productivity.

The stutterer, because of his fear of speaking and his difficulty in verbalizing in a free and spontaneous nature, disturbs the general "down-to-earth" atmosphere which is essential for good therapy. In this respect, the therapist must not be caught in the dilemma of struggling to remove the symptom primarily, but work instead with the total situation presented at the time. He must be able to go behind the stuttering as a symptom, and intercept and decode the messages the stutterer is sending by the way he presents himself in speaking, his hidden meanings, feeling tones, anxieties, inhibitions, hesitations, and especially his own word jargon.

3. To relieve the stutterer of his fears regarding change and any disturbance to his psychic equilibrium.

The stutterer lives in constant dread of having his protective structures invaded or removed, with its accompanying terror of crumbling and psychically going to pieces. The stutterer for the most part cannot face his conflicts squarely or bear their related anxiety. When he has to confront himself in a difficult speaking or other situation, he fears the consequences of the ensuing struggle and quickly retreat by stuttering and pleading helplessness.

It is essential that the stutterer be helped to face himself, to increase his tolerance for struggle, to challenge change, and to see himself less as "just a stutterer" and more as a responsible human being despite his stuttering.

What Is the Basis for Speech Techniques Used in the Treatment of Stuttering?

Those directly associated with the speech field, for the most part, feel that stuttering is a learned form of behavior; and therefore the therapy of stutterers should be one of working directly with the speech difficulty. Among some of the objectives of the techniques used are the following: (1) to weaken the forces which tend to maintain and strengthen stuttering; (2) to modify and decrease the severity of the stuttering blocks by eliminating the secondary symptoms of stuttering; (3) to help the stutterer to speak, even though he stutters, in a relatively easy and effortless fashion rather than to avoid fears and blocks; and (4) to help the stutterer in an over-all adjustment to his environment.

How Is the Technique of Voluntary Stuttering Applied?

Voluntary, or intentional, stuttering is based upon the psychological principle of negative practice. The stutterer is trained first to do intentionally what he has been doing involuntarily and unintentionally, so that he may gain control over a habit which has been controlling him. The stutterer, according to Berry and Eisenson, must learn to stutter intentionally, at first repeating his complete spasm with all the associated mannerisms. He is also encouraged to try to feel as he does in his involuntary stuttering. Aids in this procedure are the use of a mirror, which he can use to observe himself as he stutters; imitating another stutterer who, by prior arrangement, has agreed to imitate him; or attempting to imitate how he himself sounds by listening to a tape recording of his own speech.

When the stutterer has reached this stage and becomes efficient at self-imitation, he is ready for his next step in voluntary stuttering. He can now learn to repeat his evocation and be able to modify it in one or more respects decided on in advance. Normally fluent speech is not the immediate goal in this technique; rather, it is the control of stuttering through modified stuttering. Even if he feels beforehand that he can speak without stuttering, the stutterer is encouraged to pretend or fake stuttering—but to do so in a way different from his usual manner of stuttering. Finally, he is further directed to stutter easily, without struggle behavior, without blocks, and without tension, if at all possible. The objective in this form of therapy is to aid and influence the stutterer to modify and weaken his own stuttering pattern and to substitute for it a more fluent form of stuttering.

What Is Meant by Differential Relaxation in Stuttering?

Differential relaxation requires that the stutterer be able to relax one set of muscles which are to be used in a voluntary act, regardless of how tense other muscles may be. In stuttering, for instance, the major group of muscles employed are those which involve the articulatory mechanism. In the beginning, the stutterer is taught differential relaxation by encouraging an unconsciously produced tense articulatory position. He is directed to press hard, even harder than he does involuntarily, in the articulatory contact for a *t,* and to then relax the contact while he exhales so that a *t* may be produced. Following this, and soon after, the stutterer is asked to make the slightest possible contact necessary to produce a *t.* Once he can do this for one type of sound, he is given exercises to practice on other plosives, continuants, nasals, and affricates—until they are all learned. The stutterer, in this practice, has achieved his goal when he can imitate "bogey" words and feared articulatory acts with relative ease.

Finally, What Is the Adaptation Technique in the Treatment of Stuttering?

The last speech technique to be mentioned here is that known as "adaptation." Wendell Johnson and some of his associates employ the technique of repeated readings of the same material to demonstrate that the incidence of stuttering is reduced with successive readings. The underlying theoretical premise for this approach is that the occurrence of stuttering in the first reading dissipates sufficient anxiety so that there is less stuttering in successive readings. Since this has been found to be true in practice, these therapists feel that the use of this technique can demonstrate to the stutterer that, in some situations, his severe nonaffluencies can be quickly reduced and relative fluency of utterance attained. In so doing, according to this school of thought, the speech situation is changed from one conducive to stuttering to one conducive to relatively fluent speech.

Is the Removal of the Stuttering System Sufficient in the Therapy of Stuttering?

Stuttering today is no longer considered as an isolated disorder of the speech mechanism but as an outward expression of a more basic character disorganization. In a problem as complex as stuttering, any attempt toward treatment should be composite in nature and not just a rehabilitation of the speech pattern. Adequate therapy should include investigations of a medical, social, psychiatric, and re-educational nature.

Is the Use of Group Therapy of Value in the Treatment of Stuttering?

The use of group therapy is a valuable adjunct in the treatment of stuttering. It is of greatest significance when used along with, and interchangeably with, individual therapy. Alone, it would not be as effective. When individual psychotherapy can help the stutterer arrive at an understanding of his more deeply rooted conflicts, then the additional use of group therapy will give him the advantage of experiencing himself in social situations, especially in the speaking situation.

Is a Group Consisting Solely of Stutterers Successful?

Stutterers as a homogenous group tend to bog each other down in the group therapy milieu and restrict their freedom of expression and spontaneity. A heterogenous group of neurotics proved to be more alive, gave vent to more interaction, and, as a whole, much more effective therapeutically.

How Does Group Therapy Help?

The aim of the group approach in the treatment of stut-ering is threefold:

1) To break down the stutterer's old, unsound emotional reactions, habit patterns and attitudes, and to help him build up healthy, constructive new ones.

2) To overcome the patient's specific fears and anxieties, especially those regarding speech situations.

3) To foster a better social adjustment and to develop a more mature, adequate, and better-integrated personality as a whole.

What Are Some of the Suggested Ways in Which the Group Can Help in Producing Thera-peutic Results?

1) The group creates a situation in which the individual is brought face to face with himself and to experience himself as he really is. It also gives him an opportunity to act against his symptom in the specific situation that ordinarily provokes it.

2) It helps him to see that others have similar diffi-culties, conflicts, general personality traits—that he is not alone in his troubled situation. This important subjective feeling of being "in the same boat" with others ultimately adds to his own self-growth.

3) In the group situation, the stutterer can be more willing to accept his own limitations and discrepancies when he realizes that he shares them with others. It also helps him to move closer to those others in the group, and im-prove, in general, his relations to others.

4) The group enables him to express himself as freely as possible without inhibition or censorship. In so doing he can gain valuable insight into many of his defenses, ra-tionalizations, blind spots, and other aspects of his speech difficulty.

5) The group milieu gives the therapist a "real life" situation in which to observe the stutterer with his various blocks, attitudes, feelings and beliefs, especially as these factors operate in relation to others.

6) Finally, in those stutterers where resistance to change is met, the individual is much more likely to remain in therapy when he is part of a group and when he sees the progress others are making in treatment. It also gives him a realistic awareness of struggle, real suffering, and the need for sacrifices in the process toward growth.

What Might Be Considered an Ideal Therapeutic Approach to Stuttering?

A therapy program along these lines should possess all, or most, of the following characteristics:*

1) Therapy for the problem of stuttering might be viewed as a joint activity of a therapy team that includes a psychiatrist, a speech pathologist and a clinical psychologist.

2) The diagnostic evaluation of the stutterer should include attention to the vocal-mechanism centered aspects, superintended by a speech pathologist, and attention to the emotional health of the stutterer, superintended by a qualified psychiatrist. Generally, the stutterer will be administered a battery of tests, particularly projective tests by a certified clinical psychologist, that are held to be capable of throwing light on the problem of communication and on the state of emotional health of the person.

3) There should be abundant opportunities for interaction by the two therapies, with consultation at the diagnostic level, joint plannings of therapy activities, and as-

---

*Suggested by J. Villarreal in *The Psychotherapy of Stuttering,* edited by Dominick A. Barbara, M.D., 1963, Charles C Thomas, Publisher, Springfield, Illinois.

sessment that is broad enough to encourage evidences of spech fluency and evidences of emotional health as well.

Is It Possible for a Speech Therapist and a Psychiatrist to Work in the Same Therapeutic Setting?

In an experimental project begun by the author at the Karen Horney Clinic in New York City, a dynamically oriented speech therapist worked in separate meetings with the same stutterers that met with the psychiatrist in group sessions. The speech therapist's main role was to listen and gather as much information as he could regarding what was communicated by the stutterers in the group interaction. Simultaneously, there was a constant communicative interchange between myself as psychiatrist and the speech therapist. Pertinent information on what was going on which related to the work of each other was exchanged, and reactions of both therapists were evaluated intermittently.

In this experimental group, speech therapy was presented not as an isolated mechanistic phenomenon, but as a dynamic social function. Little emphasis was placed on *"what was being said,"* but on *"how it was expressed,"* *"what feelings were revealed,"* and finally, *"what effect did it produce on the stutterer."* Although some muscular retraining techniques were used to break down old disturbed speech habits, the speech therapist essentially attempted to connect this physiological impairment with those attitudes which primarily hampered it with contradictory mental sets. In so doing, the therapist not only introduced healthy precepts of real life situations, but simultaneously attempted to ameliorate the existing speech difficulty by introducing newer attitudes which could foster communication, and the ultimate freedom from stuttering.

Describe in Some Detail Doctor Bleumel's Approach to a Dynamically Speech-oriented Procedure?

The late Dr. Bleumel, a foremost authority on stuttering, formulated what he termed "basic speech reorganization." To quote from Bleumel:

> It is only in recent years that the distinction between primary and secondary stammering has been generally understood. Yet the distinction is simple, and it is one that the stammerer, in his efforts at self-help, must keep clearly in mind. The primary disorder is a blocking or muting of the mind which prevents the speaker from thinking the words clearly and saying them clearly. The secondary component is the speaker's reaction to his dilemma and his attempt to battle with it. The speaker must contend with these two components in different ways. He must recognize the fact that the secondary speech struggle is not the real difficulty. The panic, the breath-holding, the contortion, the forcing, the aversion and avoidance, the use of starters and wedges and synonyms and circumlocutions are all phases of reaction and they are not part of the primary stammering. When these reactions are recognized as secondary symptoms, they can gradually be minimized and controlled; and the stammer is then in a better position to contend with the primary speech disorder.

> The primary disturbance is the momentary blocking which effaces the mental words from the mind and leaves the speaker mute and confused. The speaker's logical recourse in this situation is to attempt to compose himself and think the words so that he can now say them—clearly and without effort. The illogical recourse is to struggle with the mouth muscles and the breathing muscles and to complicate the picture with a futile struggle reaction. This struggle must be reduced,

so that the stammerer is free to deal with his primary disturbance of muting in his inward speech. In this thinking-therapy, the speaker looks for fluency just above the ears and not just above the chin. The mind broadcasts to the mouth, and mouth gives a faithful reproduction of the verbal thinking. It gives the language that is thought, together with the inflection, the articulation, the degree of loudness, and other speech qualities that originate in the mind. There is a parallel in the matter of singing. One must think in tune in order to sing in tune; and if one is off key in singing, it is because one is off key in one's musical thinking. In speech correction, one ignores the mouth, and centers the full attention on the mind. If the mental speech is clear and concise, the oral speech will be in similar pattern and the stammering will subside.

There is another area in which the stammerer can strive for fluency; he can seek to improve the general quality of his speech quite apart from the matter of stammering. As already mentioned, facility in speech varies with different people. One man is fluent enough to become a radio commentator; another can scarcely express himself in a fully completed sentence. Thus, we see different skills in speaking just as we encounter different skills in singing; and in the case of the stammerer we find a speaker with a rather low level of verbal achievement. Quite apart from the impediment, the stammerer appears to be a non-skilled speaker; he is non-fluent; he carries a speech deficit, as it were. It was probably this non-organization of basic speech that permitted the speech function to become disorganized in early life. But the impediment being established, the frustration continued, and the speech never became organized into a pattern of normal fluency. It is true that the occasional stammerer has occasional fluency, but the fact that this fluency can be shattered by haste or emotion or stress suggests that the function of speech was never organized with any degree of security.

And here lies the stammerer's opportunity—to organize his speech even at a belated period. The procedure is to find occasion to talk in situations that offer relative fluency. This may mean talking or reading alone, reading with a partner or a study group, speaking with records or tape recordings, echoing the speech of a radio or television commentator; in fact, availing oneself of all possible opportunity of hearing and feeling one's speech in un-obstructed fluency. With the basic speech function thus improved, the stammerer is in a good position to monitor his verbal thinking in normal speech situations. He can now broadcast from the mind to the mouth with heightened self-confidence and with considerable fluency.

Do Parents of Stutterers Usually Feel Guilty about Their Children's Problem?

For the most part, the parent who is made aware that her child's stutter is basically psychological in nature is frequently distraught at the realization that she may be the cause of the difficulty and develops feelings of guilt. Unless the therapist handles this situation with skill, the parent may feel so threatened that she may be too uncomfortable to return. Parents should be handled with consideration and understanding and, whenever possible, an effort should be made to relieve them of such feelings. The parent in the interview is helped to feel that her relationship with the child might be basic to the problem and should be understood and worked through, not for the purposes of pointing the finger of guilt, but in order to determine the areas in which changes could occur so as to promote healthier emotional growth in the child. The therapist in so doing is not to be regarded as a judge or critic, but someone who can help them alleviate the conditions that are causing difficulty.

How Involved Does the Therapy of Stuttering Concern Parents?

The degree of parent treatment will depend on the severity of the total problem itself. Some cases will necessitate extensive family care and it will be necessary to treat various members of the same family. In almost every case both parents should be carefully interviewed in one or more visits. If therapy continues on a regular basis, it is also necessary to see a parent—usually the mother, who is more amenable and ready to be interviewed—at least once every other week to discuss further developments. In the parent sessions, discussions are held about the child's problems and adjustments, the parents relatedness to these problems, the situation at home which may be aggravating the problem, and anything that may be related to the child's difficulties and condition. The father, because of his many responsibilities, is limited as to time and is usually asked to see the therapist only about once a month or so. Similar discussions from his particular viewpoint occur in these interviews.

What Specific Advice Can a Therapist Give to a Parent Relating to the Handling of the Child's Stuttering?

The advice given, according to Glassner, should include the following points:

1. Do not interrogate the stuttering child.
2. During periods of stuttering, do not over-stimulate or encourage additional conversation.
3. Give the child your undivided attention when he speaks and do not interrupt him.
4. Adopt the attitude that the stuttering is time-limited and is psychologically determined.
5. Do not be critical of the child's stuttering.

6. When the child expresses concern about his speech, do not deny he is having difficulty but discuss it with him. Encourage him to discuss his reactions to this problem if he seems to want to do so.

7. Speak to the child in a calm, relaxed, well-modulated manner in order to help create a relaxed atmosphere and to give the child a good pattern to imitate.

What Can a Parent Do to Work Directly with the Speech Problem?

According to Doctor Bleumel, "the parents can do more for the non-fluent or stuttering child than all the speech clinics in the world. With the help of the parents, the child can learn to organize his speech in the comfort and security of his own home, and he can organize it into a firm and dependable function that will not later become disorganized under the impact of stress. The young child is in the natural learning period of speech and it is easy for him to learn fluency in his formative years. The child, whether a stutterer or not, should become a speech partner in the family from the first. This does not mean that conversation at the table revolves around him or is always addressed to him, but it means that he receives his share of attention; and even though he is a very, very junior member, he is addressed from time to time and he enters into the conversation with simple words that are not reduced to mere baby-talk. In this manner, the youngest member of the family can feel that he belongs, and he does not pick up his speech from fragments or leavings which his elders have discarded. The child can be made really important at the family table, and this without being spoiled. From time to time, he can be asked to chose dessert for tomorrow's dinner; and needless to say, his little ego profits from this social recognition."

Is There One Particular Kind of Therapeutic Approach to Stuttering?

The type of approach most successful is that medium through which a given child or adult who stutters can best work out his problem. Within this framework, the therapist who is well trained and who has reasonably worked through most of his own problems, and who at the same time develops his own particular techniques or skills, should have the best results. A therapist cannot expect to proceed exactly in the same manner with any two cases. The dynamics and background are never identical and the particular therapeutic approach or approaches must therefore vary. The activity to be effective must be planned around the needs of the individual stutterer based on the therapist's knowledge of the problem.

Is Play Therapy Important in the Treatment of the Child Stutterer?

Play therapy is most useful in treating all children with emotional problems because it is a permissive approach to therapy, and it permits the therapist to take part in the child's activity, helps him build a sound relationship with the child, and finally it facilitates the interpretation of the child's behavior into terms the child can understand. Theoretically, it is a psychotherapeutic approach which helps the therapist in his understanding of the child's feelings, anxieties, fantasies, while at the same time offering the child a sort of arena in which to deal with these feelings and reevaluate his personal worth at a level at which he is comfortable. Play is the child's normal medium of expression and it allows the therapist to participate in the child's world.

Should a More Immediate and Direct Approach Be Used with a Child Who Presents Marked Stuttering Manifestations?

There are some children who present such marked stuttering manifestations or are so concerned about their problem that it is necessary to give them symptomatic relief as soon as possible. This is usually done in a manner which is clear and simple at the child's level. It is usually pointed out, for instance, that with an attempt toward a general relaxation of his whole being and a willingness to become less chaotic and remain more in contact with his surroundings, the child can become less fearful and anxious, and thus feel more totally integrated.

At the speech level, relaxation can be accomplished by helping the young stutterer learn to relax the muscles of the mouth and neck, and that with a lowering of the voice, the words come out with no effort. The child will often be amazed and appear relieved to find that just by utilizing relaxed easy movements of the mouth and by not restricting the facial muscles, he has no difficulty speaking. The therapist, recommends Glassner, should demonstrate what takes place mechanistically when excessive pressure is produced within the mouth area and then illustrate how easily speech flows when there is no muscular tension. This approach can be couched in a spirit of play and the child can engage in this activity playing the "hard" and "easy" way. This technique tends to take away the overwhelming nature of the stuttering, and paves the way for further therapy and the ultimate resolution of the problem itself.

Is Drug Therapy of Value in the Treatment of Stuttering?

Drug therapy has been relatively inadequate in the young stutterer and, at best, should be used only as a supplement to other forms of treatment. In the adult, tranquilizing medications can be of some use as an adjunct to therapy in that they help diminish the degree of anxiety in the frightened, anxious, and tense person may be of some limited usefulness. Whether drugs have a specific curative value in stuttering is questionable.

What Are Some of the Indications of Improvement in Therapy?

A mere decrease in the frequency of stuttering is of little real significance. Instead, one should look to see whether there is a realistic decrease in the severity and complexity of the stuttering, and whether there is any lessening of avoidance. Other criteria of change are: (1) a general lessening of anxiety and apprehensiveness associated with speaking; (2) Whether there is a decrease in the evading of certain speech situations or certain words; (3) An increase in awareness and tolerance for frustration and struggle; (4) A total sense of inner growth, confidence, assertiveness, and a feeling of choice in the speaking situation; (5) Finally, whether he feels a greater sense of responsibility and freedom of choice in the communicative situation.

What Are Some of the Indications of Resistance to Therapy?

Among the indications of little change to therapy are:
1. No reduction in complexity or severity of stuttering.
2. No reduction in fear or concern for the stuttering itself.
3. Continued avoidance reactions, "bugaboo" words and substitutions.
4. No real initiative, motivation, or sense of struggle before or during stuttering.

5. Obvious signs of alienation, resignation, inertia, passivity and hopelessness.

Is the Increase of the Stuttering Itself a Poor Sign in Therapy?

Not necessarily. The increase of stuttering at certain intervals in therapy usually indicates that some more of the stutterer's protective structures are being invaded upon, and that the individual may merely be daring to open himself more in the speaking situation. It may also indicate a testing of the therapist in the form of a plea on helplessness, and a need to return to a more protective and dependent position. When this happens, the therapist should not "pull at his stutterer" nor disturb too forcibly the "status quo." Instead, he should be patient, understanding, and have a real feeling for the stutterer's dilemma. At the same time, the therapist should not encourage the stutterer to make unrealistic claims on his "helplessness," but should remain firm, consistent and affirmative throughout.

How Is the Termination of Treatment in the Stuttering Child Evaluated?

The termination of treatment must be a carefully planned procedure. When it is agreed that the child is stuttering less and that he is functioning well in other life situations, the frequency of the visits is reduced. This modified weaning process continues until the child is able to spend longer and longer periods of time without treatment, until he becomes and remains symptom free. After the child has been free from stuttering and other compulsive behavior for approximately three months, a discussion is held with the child and the parents included, and the case is dismissed. In most instances, as the child feels his own inner growth, he will be able to indicate his own progress and the desire to terminate therapy.

How Is the Termination of Treatment in the Adult Stutterer Determined?

To be effective, the therapeutic situation should give the adult stutterer what he most surely needs, i.e.,—a sense of belonging, an atmosphere of unity and union, a feeling of respect with others, and finally a controlled environment where he is able to act out his symptom to his best interests.

As the therapy progresses, the stutterer usually becomes more realistic, and along with this there is also a con-comitant and gradual lessening or removal of the symptom of stuttering. As he comes out of his neurotic web, and feels greater spontaneity and inner freedom, he will also be-come less driven and compulsive. He will progressively block less as a total individual, become less inhibited and more flexible, leading simultaneously to a decrease in hesi-tant, blocking and stuttering speech.

In the final analysis, the person who stutters must give up many illusions of himself, and ultimately tend to discard his image of himself as "a perfect speaker." In his growth toward emotional security, he begins to healthily re-evalu-ate and re-orientate many of his attitudes and values to-ward life. The more adequate a person he becomes, the more balanced will his verbalizations become. The stutterer can now feel less dependency upon the opinions of his audience, have a greater sense of self-worth, and take more responsibility for himself, even when he speaks. He will learn to feel and experience his words and expressions as his own, coming from within himself, and will have the courage to stand behind his own individual assertions and convictions. The more inner strength he feels, the more solid ground he will feel beneath him, and less inadequate will he present himself in all circumstances, including that of verbal communication. As he hides less behind his de-fenses, and comes out more into the open, he will assume a more honest front, and he will as a result have much less need to stutter. With adequate therapy, he will in the end result tend to discard his neurosis and all that it implies— including that of stuttering.

How Can the Family Physician Be of Help to Parents of Stutterers?

The physician's first step is referral to a psychiatrist, a speech therapist or clinic. Moreover, it should be emphasized that the sooner therapy is begun, the better is the prognosis. Stuttering is not something a child *"grows out of."* Rather, it is a disorder he "grows into."

To parents who fear stuttering, the physician should emphasize the fact that hesitations and non-fluencies are normally present in every child. However, if with parents who present a persistent anxiety or concern about their child's speech, the problem "should not be ignored," but referred to a qualified specialist in this field. A few consultations at this level could easily ameliorate the situation and avoid the development of a more serious problem.

Parents of stutterers should be reminded that the young stutterer requires regular checkups. Good diet and adequate rest are essential. Fatigue increases frequency of stuttering and parents should be advised that their children require earlier bedtimes and more rest than other children. Also, they should be informed that the emotional tension in children who stutter might give rise to toilet and feeding habits.

Finally, the parent should be educated to her child's tendency toward awkwardness, clumsiness, and poor motor coordination. Also, that he often feels inadequate and may tend toward introverted behavior, avoiding speaking situations where he will meet with disapproval. The family physician can help by advising family, friends, and teachers of the stutterer's special problem. Above all, the speech difficulty should not be ignored, and as many tensions and anxiety-producing elements as possible should be eliminated from his environment.

Where Might One Find Professional Help?

In every single case of suspected or beginning stuttering which does not stop within a short period of time, fully qualified professional consultation should be obtained. You may obtain information concerning qualified psychiatrists or psychologists specializing in speech and hearing problems from your nearest office of the American Psychiatric or Psychological Association. Today, there are many speech clinics in universities, hospitals, and various rehabilitation centers serving children and adults. The American Speech and Hearing Association will provide you with information concerning the location of clinics and clinicians. Its address is: 1001 Connecticut Avenue, N. W., Washington 6, D.C.

INDEX